Dad,
It was ~~~~~ful
to have you visit.
Come again soon & bring
Judy too!

how to be
HAPPY,
dammit

XOXO

January 3?

P.S. Thank you so much
for all the help.
The yard & (TREES) look
beautiful!

how to be

HAPPY,
dammit

a cynic's guide to spiritual happiness

karen salmansohn

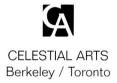

CELESTIAL ARTS
Berkeley / Toronto

A Kirsty Melville Book

Celestial Arts
an imprint of Ten Speed Press
PO Box 7123
Berkeley, California 94707
www.tenspeed.com

Distributed in Australia by Simon and Schuster Australia, in Canada by Ten Speed Press
Canada, in New Zealand by Southern Publishers Group, in South Africa by Real Books, and
in the United Kingdom and Europe by Publishers Group UK.

Concept and book packaging by Amazon Girl, Inc.
Design by zinzell – www.zinzell.com

Library of Congress Cataloging-in-Publication Data
Salmansohn, Karen.
    How to be happy, dammit : a cynic's guide to spiritual happiness /
Karen Salmansohn.
        p. cm.
    ISBN-13: 978-1-58761-119-3 (pbk.)
    ISBN 1-58761-119-8 (pbk.)
    1. Happiness.   I. Title.
    BJ1481 .S285   2001
    170'.44—dc21   2001028596

Printed in China

16 17 18 19 – 12 11 10 09 08

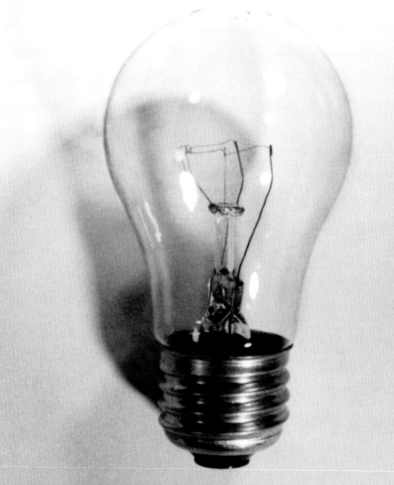

THE IDEA FOR THIS BOOK:
To create the first and only self-help book that merges Psychology, Biology, Eastern Philosophy, Western Philosophy, Quantum Physics, and the Zen of Bazooka Joe that's guaranteed to perk up even the most cynical spirit.

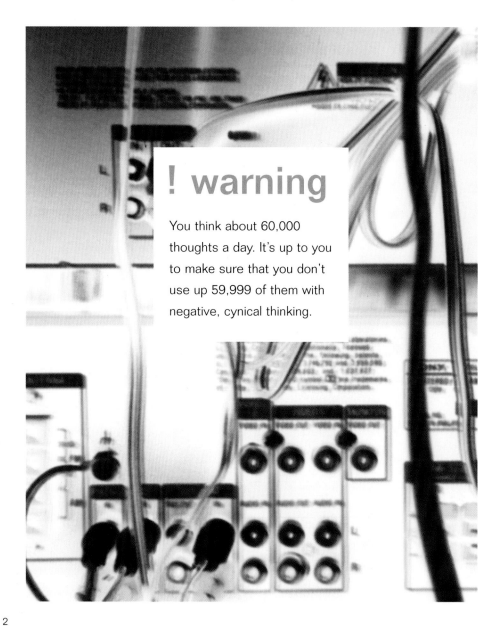

! warning

You think about 60,000 thoughts a day. It's up to you to make sure that you don't use up 59,999 of them with negative, cynical thinking.

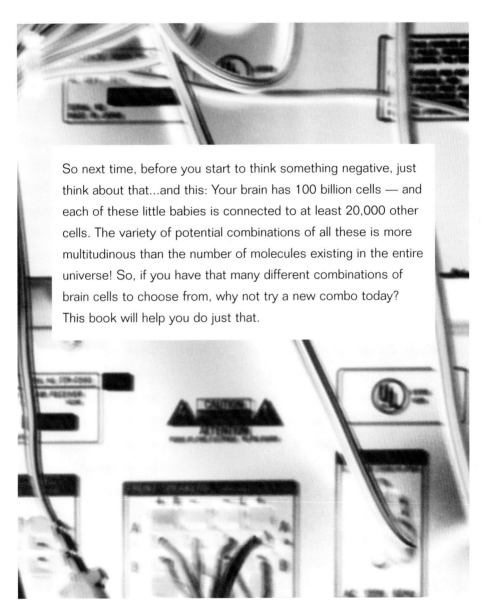

So next time, before you start to think something negative, just think about that...and this: Your brain has 100 billion cells — and each of these little babies is connected to at least 20,000 other cells. The variety of potential combinations of all these is more multitudinous than the number of molecules existing in the entire universe! So, if you have that many different combinations of brain cells to choose from, why not try a new combo today? This book will help you do just that.

Read on...

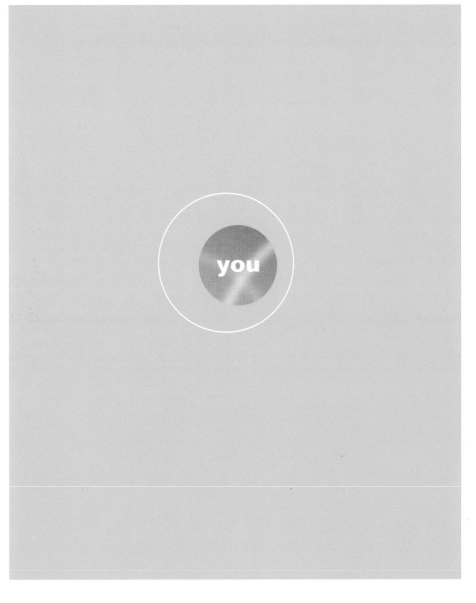

You are born into this world an innocent.

Guilt-free.
Sugar-free.
Caffeine-free.

You are noble and pure.

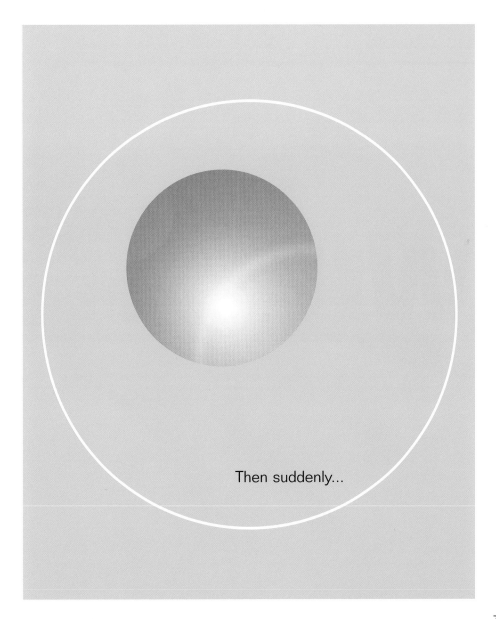

Then suddenly...

WHACK.

You are spanked.
Really hard.
This is unfair.
You have done nothing wrong.
You know this for a fact.

How?

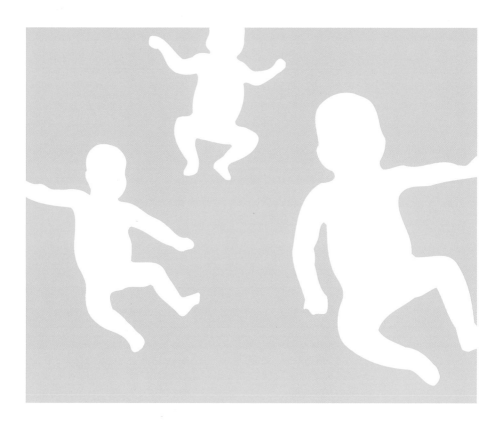

You haven't had time to do anything — period.
You are only 3 1/2 seconds old.

You haven't had time to catch your breath, let alone time to covet a neighbor
or furtively screen calls on your answering machine. You don't even have an
answering machine yet. You don't even have people to avoid yet — you are
that spanking new.

Which brings us back to that spanking.

WHY?

Why you?

Why all the pain?

Although you're only 3 1/2 seconds old, you have just been taught a

big life lesson.

ARE
YOU
PAYING

ATTENTION YET?

#1

Pain exists.

Life can hurt.

Like a lot.

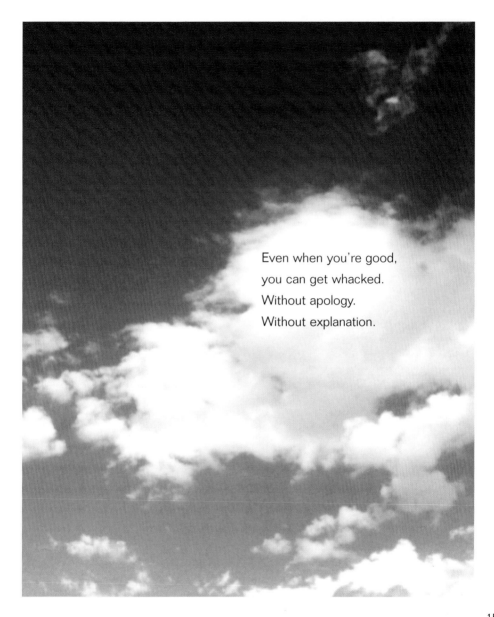

Even when you're good,
you can get whacked.
Without apology.
Without explanation.

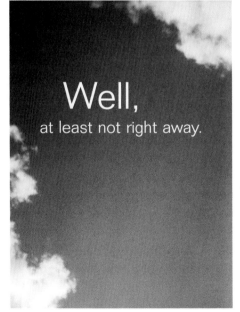

Well,
at least not right away.

It's not until later, that you finally

learn...

LIFE LESSON #2

That pain back in LIFE LESSON #1 was for your benefit.

You were being
taught to breathe,
invited to suck
down a yummy
oxygen/nitrogen
cocktail. That
painful whack
was necessary
for your growth.

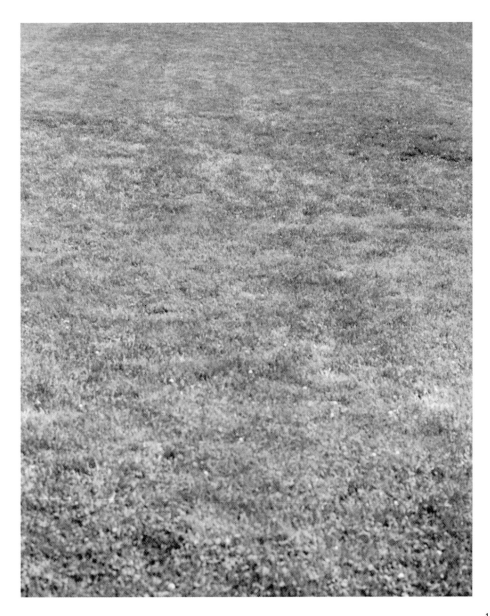

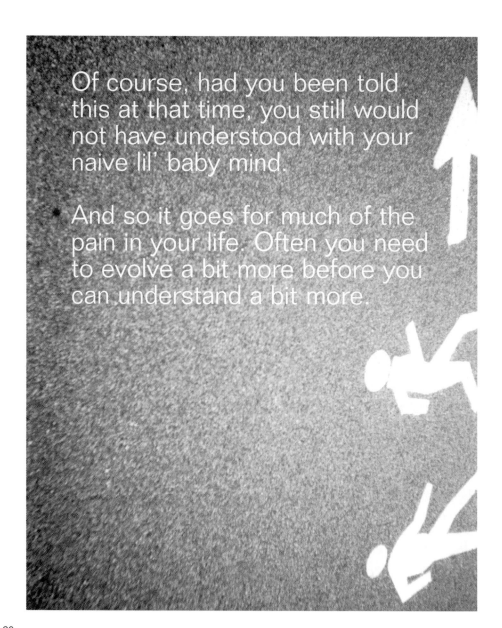

Of course, had you been told this at that time, you still would not have understood with your naive lil' baby mind.

And so it goes for much of the pain in your life. Often you need to evolve a bit more before you can understand a bit more.

By now you know:

you live in a world of 1,000,001 interpretations.

By now you know:

you must resist staying stuck on merely 1.

Which brings you to...

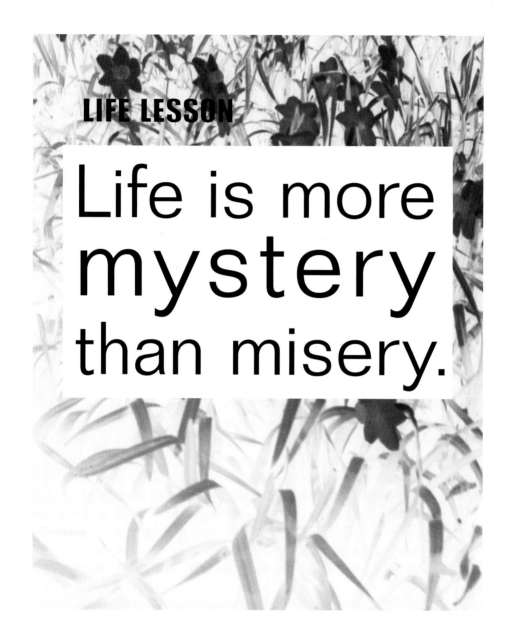

LIFE LESSON

Life is more mystery than misery.

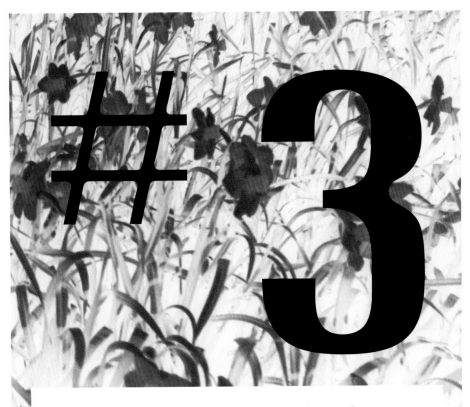

#3

In time, insights take form.

You relate to that expression:

"No pain, no gain."

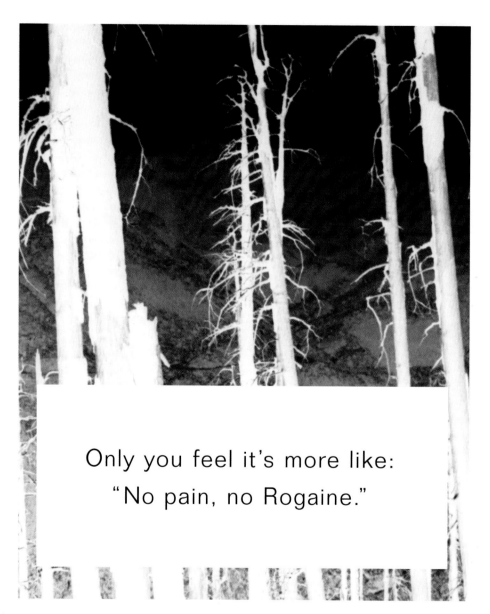

Only you feel it's more like:

"No pain, no Rogaine."

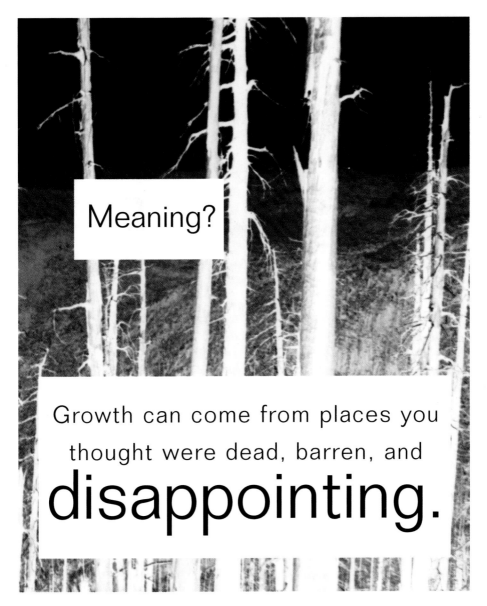

Meaning?

Growth can come from places you thought were dead, barren, and **disappointing.**

Which leads to you to...

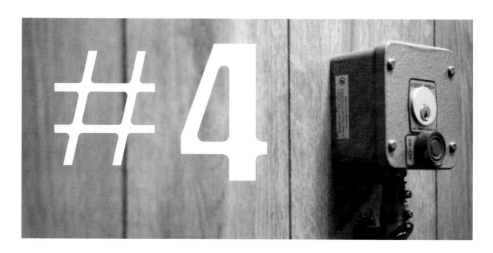

You always have a choice of emotional responses to life.

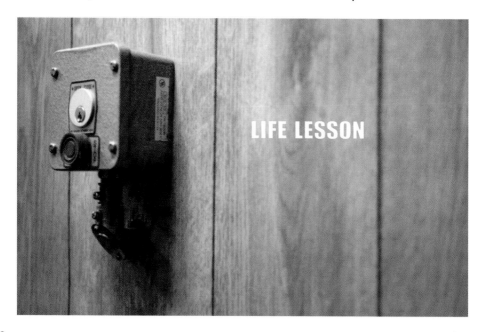

LIFE LESSON

Happiness

is not about what happens to you, but how you choose to respond to what happens. That's why it's called happiness not happenness — though it could be called hope-ness. You must always leave room for hope that all has happened for good cause.

Or to quote the philosopher Arthur Schopenhauer:

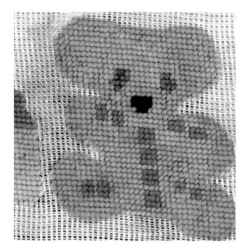

Life may be compared to a piece of embroidery of which, during the first half of our time, we get a sight of the right side, and during the second half, of the wrong.

"

The wrong side is not as pretty...

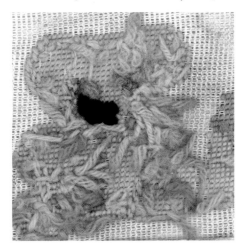

but it is more instructive; it shows the way in which the threads have been worked

together [to make the pattern].

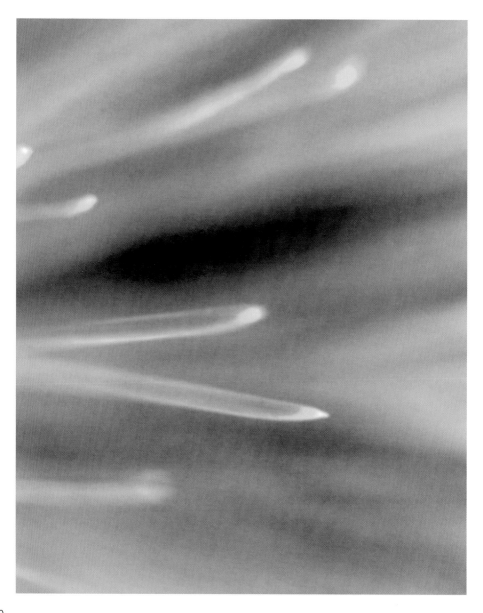

You feel this Arty guy's got it pretty right.

What he says reminds you of a tip your gardener friend told you...

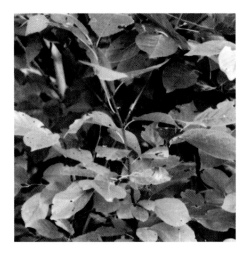

"

Some plants are only meant to last for a certain season or a certain time, (said your gardener friend).

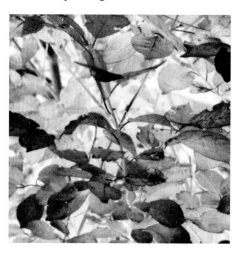

If you try to make them live longer, you will be a bad gardener.

You were struck by how the same goes for people and jobs, how sometimes it seems people and jobs — and/or problems in general — are brought into your life for certain reasons, to stay around for a certain time, to teach you certain things.

Of this you are certain.

For instance, they've taught you...

LIFE LESSON

Judge a tree by its fruits. And ditto for people.

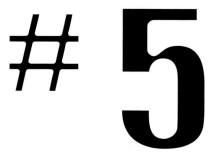

You can always tell who someone is by the circumstances they grow. The apple doesn't fall far from the tree — and neither does the bad banana.

By now you know...to avoid bad banana people.

And you especially know it's fruitless to ask bad banana people for advice. For instance, don't ask career-less people for career advice...or relationship-less people for relationship advice.

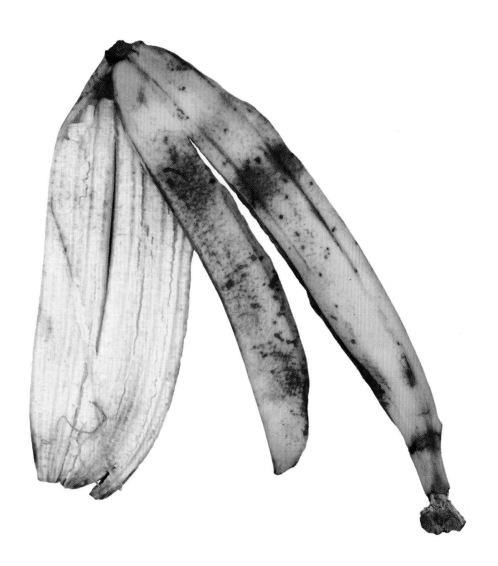

Which brings you to…

LIFE LESSON

#6

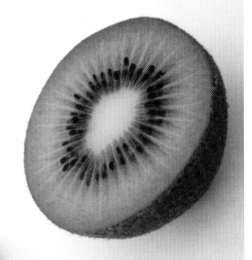

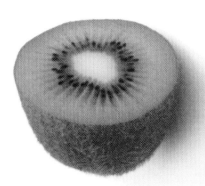

Never go shopping for kiwis in a shoe store.

Some people just don't have what you need. So why waste time,
banging on their doors, ringing their bells, demanding service?

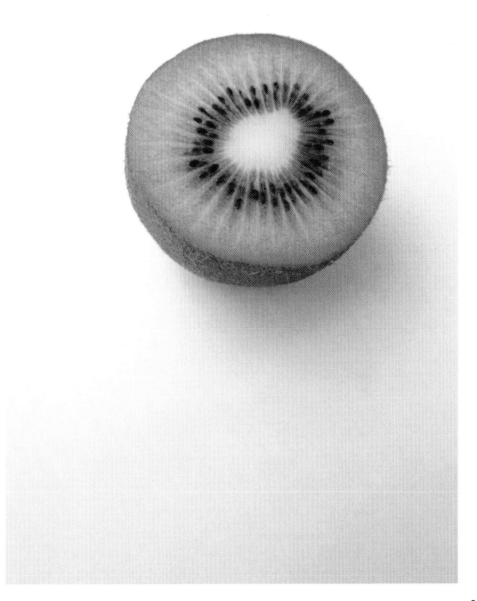

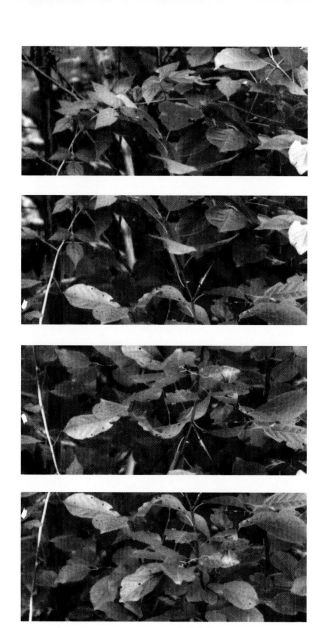

When you think about the kiwi-less people in your life, you're reminded of yet another wise thing your gardener friend told you — this time about a dying purple plant you once had in your home. You had been keeping this purple plant in direct sunlight, feeding it plenty of water, spoiling it silly. However, rather than blossom at your touch, it was perishing. When you asked your gardener friend about it, he chuckled and explained: "This breed of plant thrives best in darkness — with very little water." You were surprised. You had thought that all plants craved lots of water and lots of sunlight. Now you know: some need less to live on, some crave being left alone. And the same goes for people.

Which brings you to...

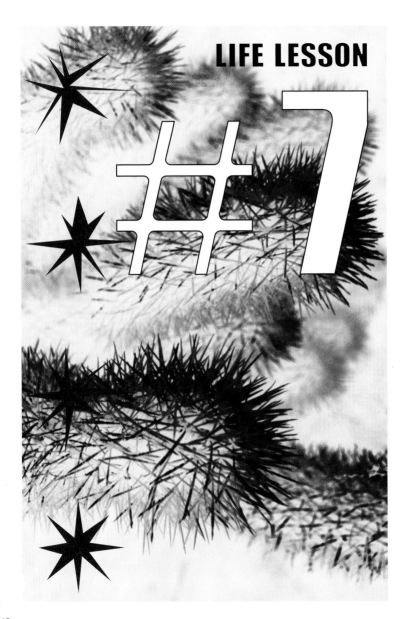

LIFE LESSON #7

You — and those you've
befriended/worked with/slept
with — each of you — just
like plants — comes with your
own unique feeding manual.
You each have your own
needs and speeds for growth.
You must read each person's
instruction manual carefully —
then proceed with caution!

Which brings you to...

#8

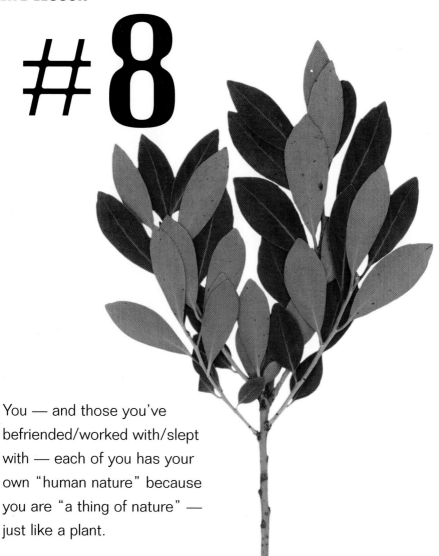

You — and those you've befriended/worked with/slept with — each of you has your own "human nature" because you are "a thing of nature" — just like a plant.

And just like a plant, you
too are governed by the
same laws of nature.

It's like this:

We all come from the same Big
Bubbling Pot of World Primordial
Nature Stew. Because of this,
you are governed — along with
your Pot Mates (like plants and
flowers and bananas) — under
the same Laws of...

Primordial Nature.

These laws include the ever popular:

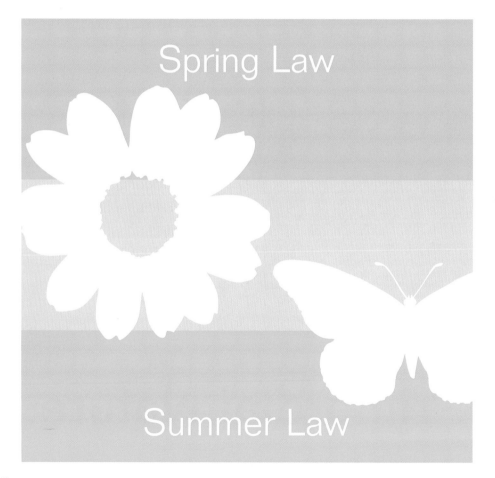

Spring Law

Summer Law

You have tried your best to break these four laws...

but they've been more successful at breaking you.

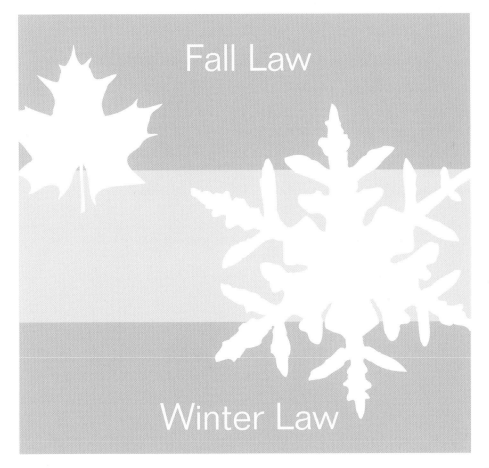

Fall Law

Winter Law

For instance, at some point in your year (every year) it seems your life hits a "winter phase" of coldness and darkness with very little growth and fertility — a phase that gets you thinking:

Oh no.
That's it, my life is over.
Everything good
is gone.

The world sucks.

Only to find that...whaddayaknow...

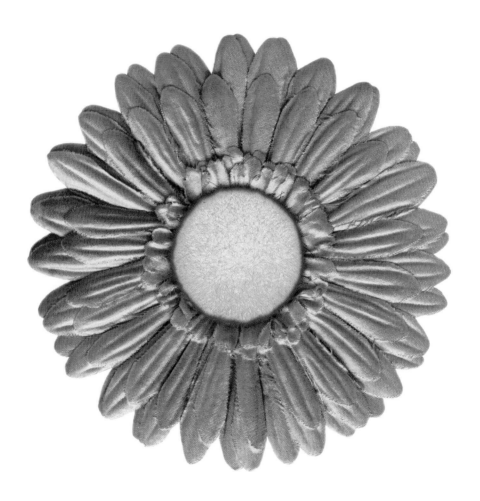

your winter phase ends and the Spring Law arrives to spring you free into a phase filled with renewal and growth and brightness. Then comes your summer phase, followed by your fall phase, followed by winter, spring, summer, etc...etc...

LIFE LESSON

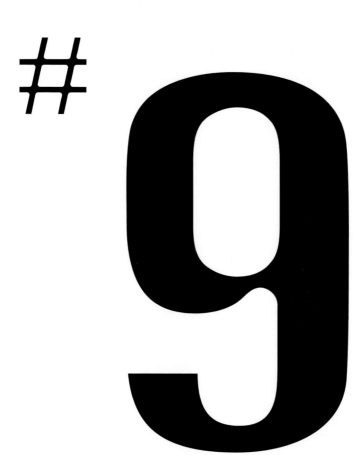

THE ONLY CONSTANT IS CHANGE.

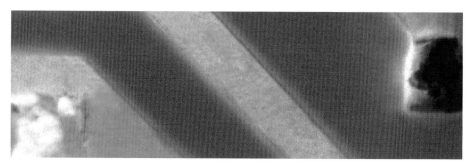

AND THINGS
CAN CHANGE AT ANYTIME
LIKE THIS TYPEFACE
OR THIS LANGUAGE... VOILA. SI!
BØRGKP MJPO?
INTO A LANGUAGE YOU
CANNOT UNDERSTAND.
YOUR WORST FEAR:
NOT UNDERSTANDING.
ALTHOUGH YOU KNOW, THAT...

YOU KNOW?

#6

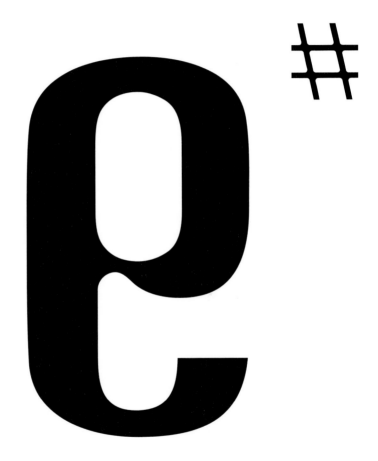

YOU NEVER KNOW.

Which reminds you of a good symbolic fable...

A GOOD SYMBOLIC FABLE IN A BOX

"Dope On a Rope"

This criminal had committed a crime. (Because hey, that's what criminals do. That's their job.) Anyway, he was sent to the king for his punishment. The king told him he had a choice. He could be hung by a rope or take the punishment behind the big dark scary steel door. The criminal quickly decided on the rope. As the noose was being slipped on him, he asked, "Out of curiosity, what's behind that door?" The king laughed and said, "You know, it's funny, I offer all you guys the same choice, and nearly all of you pick the rope." "So," said the criminal, "what's behind the door? Obviously, I won't tell anyone," he said, pointing to the noose around his neck. The king paused then answered, "Freedom, but it seems most people are so afraid of the unknown that they immediately take the rope."

You relate. You know.

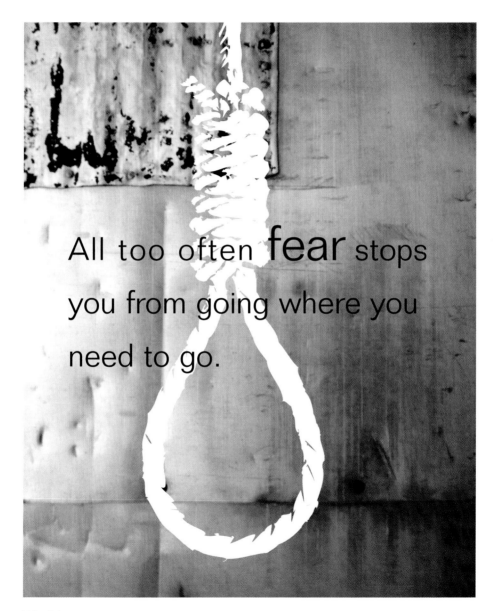

All too often **fear** stops you from going where you need to go.

LIFE LESSON #10

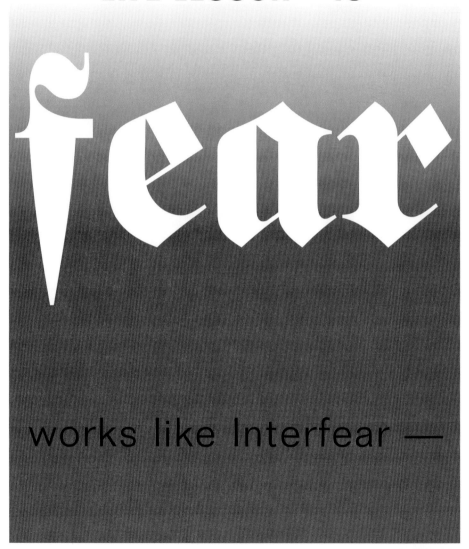

fear

works like Interfear —

stopping you from getting what you really want/need.

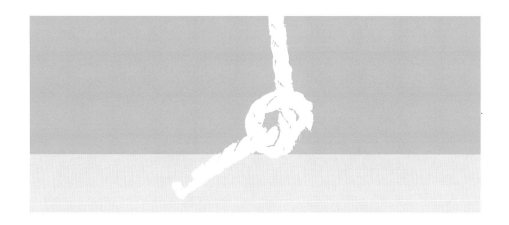

All too often you have to be at the end of your rope to be tempted to move through your fear...

and go for the unfamiliar, the unknown,

to change.

LIFE LESSON # 11

If you keep doing what you've always been doing, then you'll keep getting what you've always been getting.

You must courageously
break the habit of your
habits, or every year you
will be doomed to live out:
"Same #$%&!. Different
Outfit." The style of your
clothes may change, but
the style of your circum-
stances won't.

Which reminds you of a story...

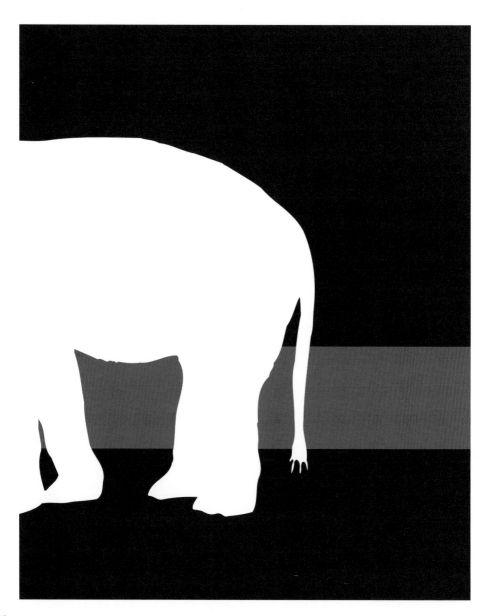

"The Elephant Truly Never Forgets"

The first trick an elephant trainer teaches an elephant is not to escape. When the elephant is still but a baby, the trainer chains the infant's leg to a huge log, so when/if the elephant tries to escape, the log proves stronger and he gives up. Eventually the elephant becomes so used to its captivity, that even when it has grown huge and strong, all the trainer has to do is merely tie the chain around the elephant's leg to anything — even a tiny little twig — and the elephant won't even try to escape.

It has become a prisoner of its past.

This elephant and its twig remind you
of you and your childhood. Though you
believe childhood habits can be broken.
You say: childhood shmildhood. In fact,
you often feel yours was more of a
"shmildhood." And your parents were
often more like "shmarents."

But, so what?

That was then. This is now. Time has passed. You can let go. Move on....Can't you?

Yes, you can...

step back from that twig!

The trick is: you must first see it's only a silly lil' twig.

Which brings you to...

#12

In order to see the
path to what you
want, you must first
see clearly what is

holding you back.

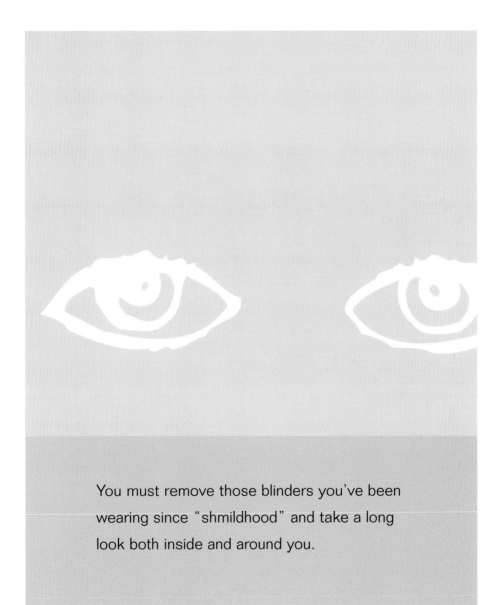

You must remove those blinders you've been wearing since "shmildhood" and take a long look both inside and around you.

BUT...

at first you feel it's
safer — healthier —
for these blinders to
remain on. So much
so, you confuse
these blinders for
Band-Aids.

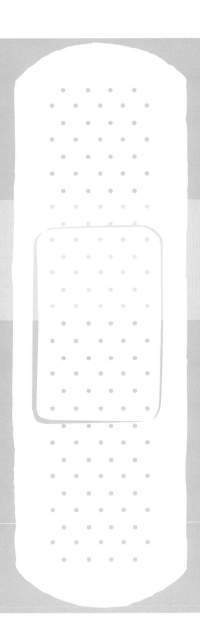

Band-Aids
that can
heal you.

But you are
wrong.

These Pseudo
Band-Aids won't
heal you.

(ouch)

Unfortunately you are also afraid to remove these Pseudo Band-Aids because you believe it will hurt a lot to remove them — which is true. But this pain won't last for long — and it (ironically) will be your true and only path to healing.

Which brings you to...

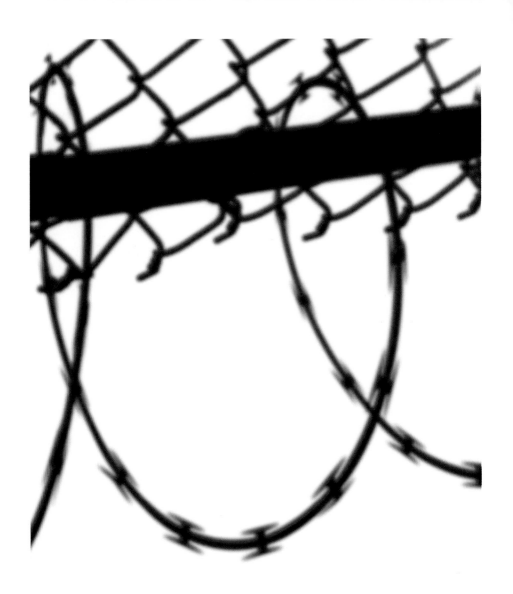

\# 13

LIFE LESSON

If you want to change your life,
you must first be ready to see
and feel some

painful truths...

Like...

Boy, have I been leading the life of an idiot — that's only a teeny lil' twig. In fact, I put the I into Idiot...

And who wants to see that?

Not you.

You like to see yourself as 100% Superman, with 0% Clark Kent.

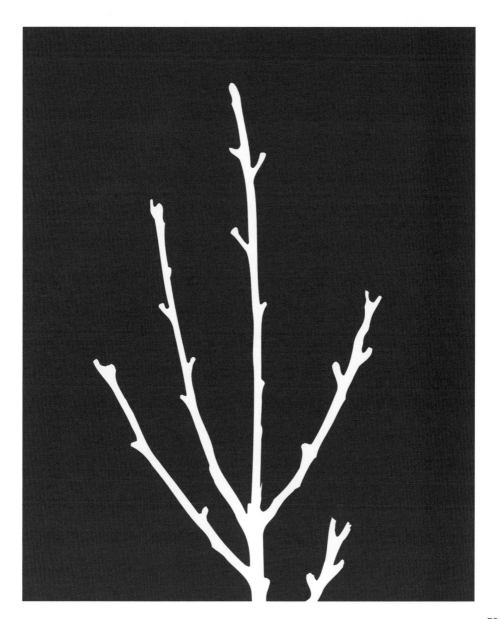

79

Your problem?

You are both.

But in your version of this Superman/Clark Kent story, you walk around in your Superman outfit...and meanwhile, in your secret identity, you are really the fearful, wimpy Clark Kent.

You've foolishly tried to increase your super power status by improving upon your tights — making them flashier, ritzier — and on occasion flinging your cape in other people's faces. Meanwhile, it's your weak Clark Kent secret self that needs the bolstering.

Otherwise, all you'll ever be is a wimp in fancy tights who can't fly.

Which reminds you of another story...

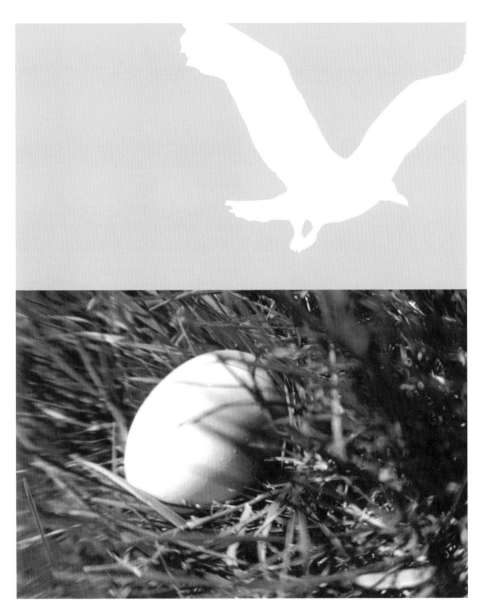

"Which Came First: The Eagle or the Egg?"

A little boy was wandering in the forest and came upon an eagle's nest. He plucked an egg, brought it back to his farm, and giggling to himself, slid it under a mama-to-be chicken. Soon after, this chicken's eggs hatched, and there among the chicklets was a female eaglette. This little eaglette grew up with her chicken peers, learning all sorts of chicken habits: how to walk like a chicken, squawk like a chicken, eat like a chicken. This eagle did it all. However, no matter how passionately she put her all into her chicken existence, she always felt something was missing. She didn't know what, but she felt an inner emptiness. One day she looked up in the sky and saw a beautiful bird, soaring freely among the clouds. She felt this pang of awe mixed with a weird sense of connection. She longed to be up there flying, too. Suddenly, she had this flash of insight. She flapped her wings and to her surprise, took off. That's when she realized that all along there was more to her than mere chickenhood. She was meant to fly — as well as cash in on some other pretty nifty eagle perks.

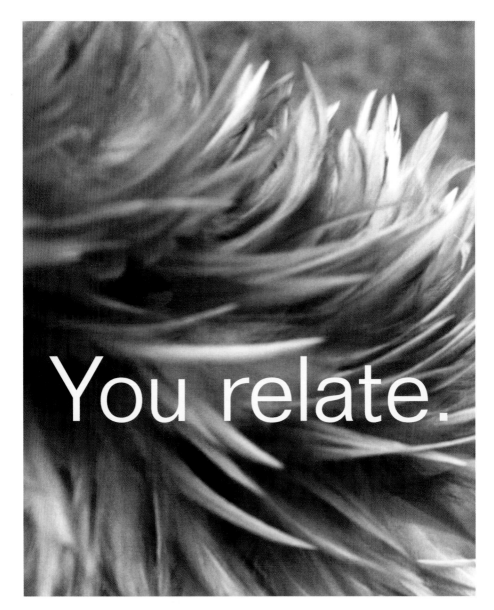

Often you feel you are an eagle leading the life of a mere chicken.

— or working with a chicken.

— or sleeping with a chicken.

Although you know: eagles are fearless. Chickens live up to their name "chicken" — and live by fear.

And you know: an eagle's first step to living the life of an eagle is to face all fears.

And an eagle's first and #1 fear is: "What will my chicken friends think if I start to live differently?"

Which brings you to...

#14

You must declare your own Independence Day, then your own Independence Year, then your own Independence Life. The purpose of your life is to find the purpose of your life.

This means: you must listen to your heart, listen to your belly, listen to NPR — but you must stop listening to your shmarents and your shmriends. (After all, just look at their crazy fruit trees!)

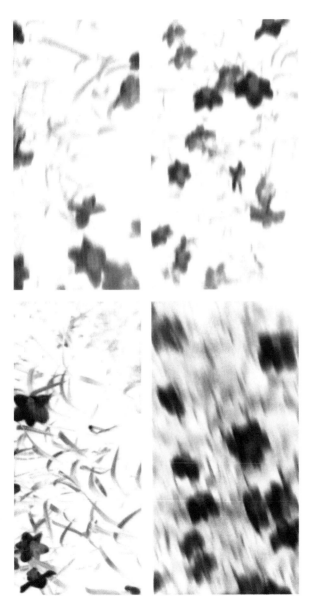

You realize: being who you want to be, and doing what you want to do, is self-respect. But that's not all, folks. It's also one of your Pot of Primordial Stew Club Membership Duties. Something even your Pot Mate the flower knows to wisely cash in on. A flower instinctively goes toward the light. It doesn't spend time worrying if people will mistake it for a weed or if it's taking too much sun. It wisely and simply follows its primal flower gut instincts to attain its highest level of flowerosity.

Conversely, you — and your busy, busy brain —

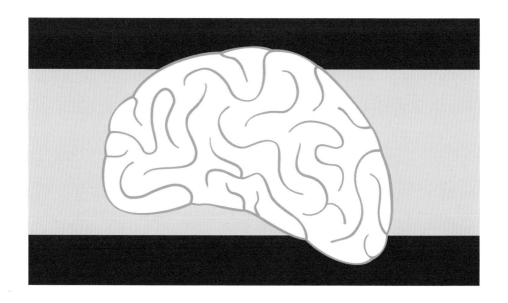

have been programmed to think, think, think —
and so you have been ignoring your heart's
instincts. Just like that eagle in its chicken
days.

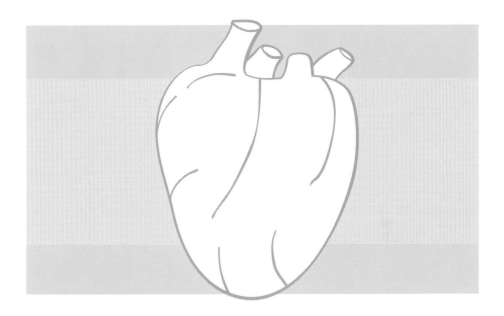

It's when that eagle finally followed its heart
that her life finally began to soar.

Which brings you to...

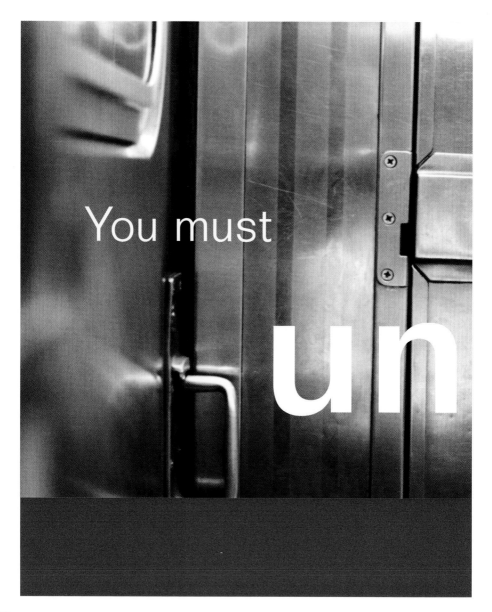

You must un

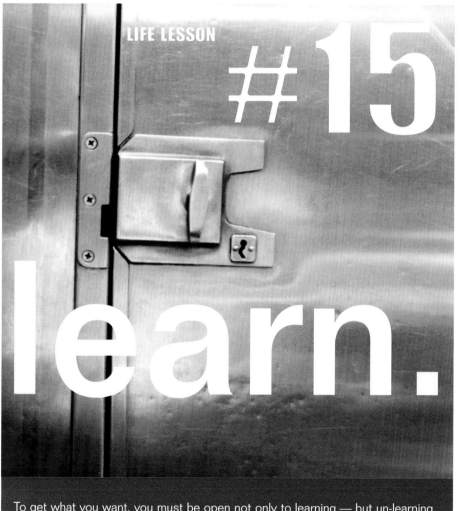

#15

learn.

To get what you want, you must be open not only to learning — but un-learning. You must sign up for un-lessons — where you un-learn learned fear, guilt, anger, jealousy, insecurity — and that's just for starters.

In other words, before you write your to-do list of
what you want, you have to write your to un-do list
and your to-don't list. So you get a piece of paper
and you write down the following six categories:
money, love, sex, family, power, happiness. Next
to each of these categories you write down your
negative views — your fears, your guilts, your
insecurities — that you must un-learn and un-feel.

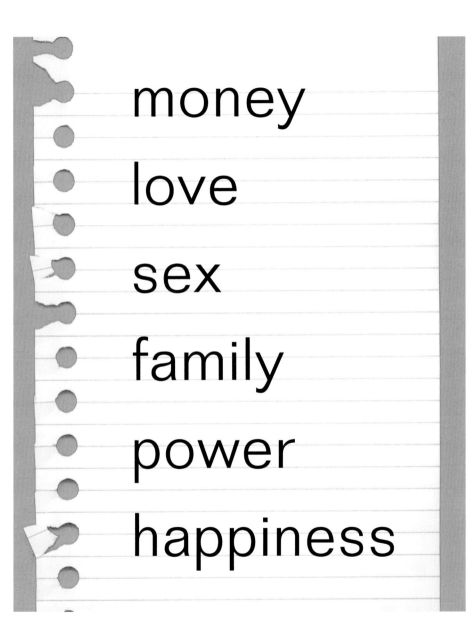

money

love

sex

family

power

happiness

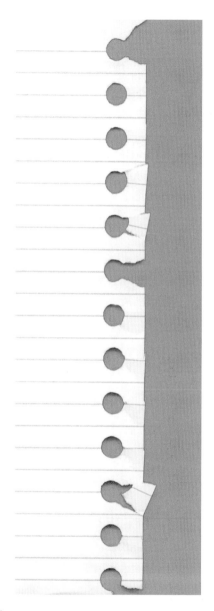

For instance, you ask yourself what negative views you have about money. Like: Do you believe all rich people are superficial jerks — hence if you become rich you too might become a superficial jerk? Do you suffer from Keeping Down with the Joneses syndrome? Do you feel guilty about surpassing your friends — and/or parents — in wealth? If so, you must un-learn and un-feel these negative ideas and negative emotions....And you find that when you trade in these negative beliefs and emotions for positive ones, you start getting more in harmony with receiving money. You start seeing money everywhere.

Even in the word *harmony*, which suddenly now looks to you like *harmoney*.

OK...

Let's say you are capable of finding these negative emotions...but unsure how to truly lose them once you've found them. What then?

How can you truly make sure you un-learn and un-feel all your negativity?

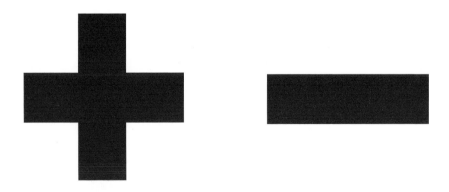

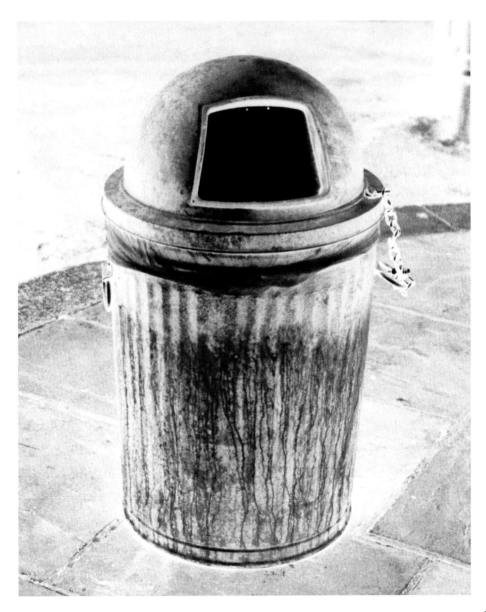

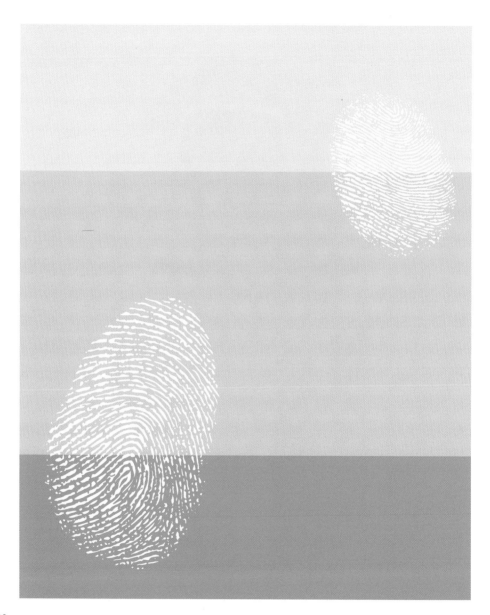

The answer: play a little game called "Find the Meaning in Life's Past Meannesses."

In part ONE of this game, you "Return to the Scene of the Crime" and playact detective. You track down your most bad, dark, depressing — grumble/grumble/grumble — childhood (and even recent) memories that led to your original negative beliefs and emotions.

In part TWO of this game, you "Return to the Scene of the Sublime." Now you must playact Hollywood screenwriter and find the meaning in your suffering. You must rewrite these events so you see them as something positive — just like a Hollywood screenwriter generously allows his fictional movie characters to eventually — clunk! Oh yeah! — see the fortune in their misfortune by story's end!

Which brings you to...

#16

This is the secret to happiness — in 3 words:

1. rationalize

2. rationalize

3. rationalize

You find it's helpful to lie to yourself about your past pain...and all the rotten things that have happened to you. And it's only fair — since everyone else is lying to you too anyway. Just kidding. Sort of. Well, achem, remember this is a cynic's guide to spiritual happiness.

You decide to see...

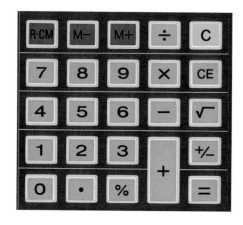

equals.

Your enemies = your teachers. Your
failure = your wisdom. Your mistakes =
your lucky discoveries. Your conflicts =
your growth opportunities. Your undesired
endings = your desirable beginnings. Your
grapes of wrath = your raisons d'etre.
Your painful feelings = your proud proof
that you are dealing with your feelings —
head on!

And there's a freebee bonus benefit to doing the above...

You begin to be less judgmental about your:

rage, fear, pain, conflicts, and disappointments...

not only for what has happened in the past but

also when it comes to your present and future.

Which brings you to...

LIFE LESSON # 17

You must celebrate Non-Judgment Day, then Non-Judgment Year, then **Non-Judgment Life.**

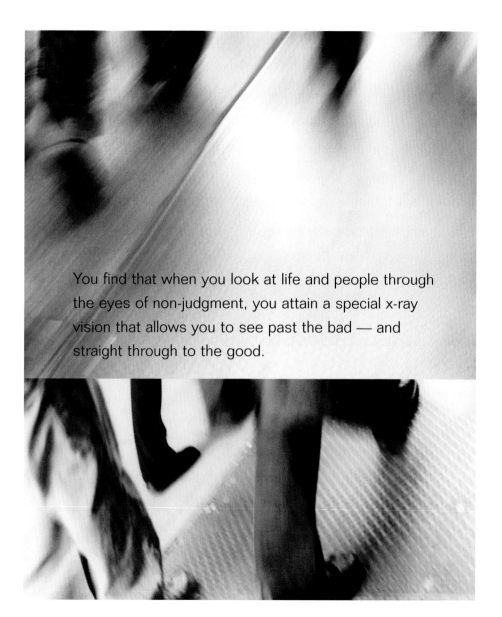

You find that when you look at life and people through the eyes of non-judgment, you attain a special x-ray vision that allows you to see past the bad — and straight through to the good.

Which leads you to...

LIFE LESSON

18

You must relax and

enjoy the ride.

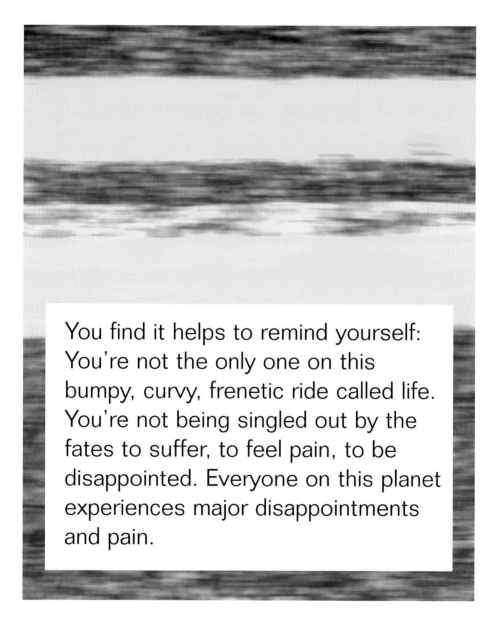

You find it helps to remind yourself: You're not the only one on this bumpy, curvy, frenetic ride called life. You're not being singled out by the fates to suffer, to feel pain, to be disappointed. Everyone on this planet experiences major disappointments and pain.

Every member of the Fortune 500 Club

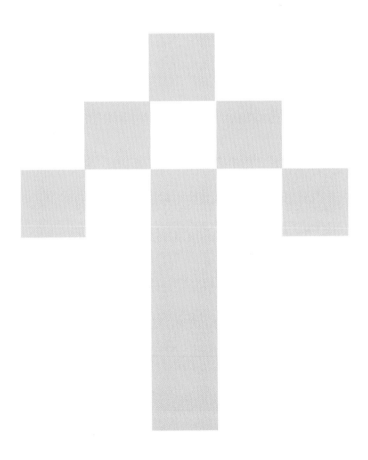

could also be eligible for membership in the

Misfortune 500 Club.

The only difference between these two clubs is: those very successful people who are members of the Fortune 500 Club know that when/if you fall on your face, you must use the leverage to bounce back higher.

Which brings you to...

#19

LIFE LESSON

You must not live in denial that disappointment and failure and pain and conflict and darkness and evil exist — they are out there.

Every silver lining always has its cloud.

This is a world of duality: of good and bad, yin and yang, decaffeinated and caffeinated. So you must always be prepared!

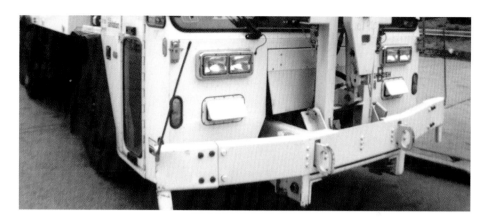

It's like this:

If you didn't accept that Good Humor Trucks existed, then you'd risk getting run over by one someday. Well, the same goes with those "Bad Humor" Trucks that are dangerously careening around out there. You also know that just because Bad Humor Trucks exist, does not mean you must walk around constantly looking for fleets of them — or else you'll never be able to get anywhere — and you'll miss out on the now.

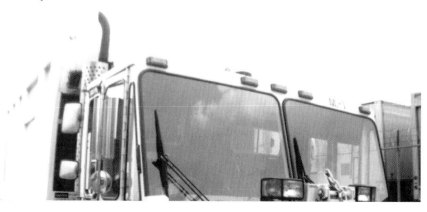

Which brings you to...

LIFE LESSON

20

You must have Great Non-Expectations.

It's self-defeating living in a tense future tense, second-guessing, third-guessing, 158th-guessing life.

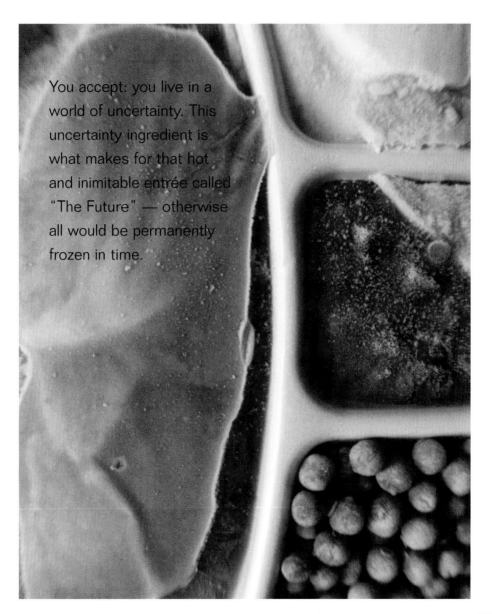

You accept: you live in a world of uncertainty. This uncertainty ingredient is what makes for that hot and inimitable entrée called "The Future" — otherwise all would be permanently frozen in time.

You realize uncertainty affects everyone and everything on this planet — right down to teeny-weeny electrons. You've heard even your Local Quantum Physicist cannot predict the future of pet laboratory electrons when they are let loose in experiments. Sometimes these electrons live the life of a wave, sometimes a particle — one never knows, which can be very unsettling.

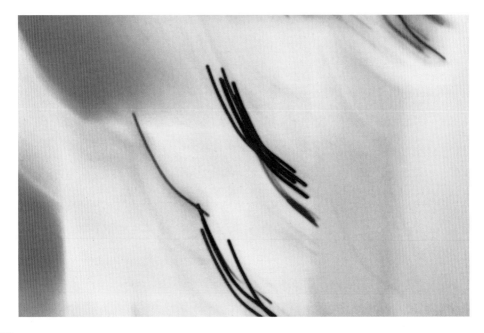

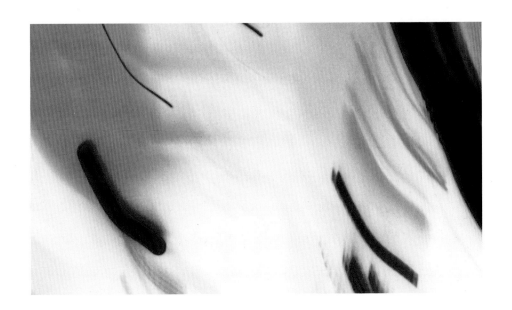

You realize that if even a smart Quantum Physicist can't predict the future of an electron — one of the teeniest particles found in this vast universe — then you are no better off trying to lay down bets on that bigger and lumpier chunk of the universe called "Your Life."

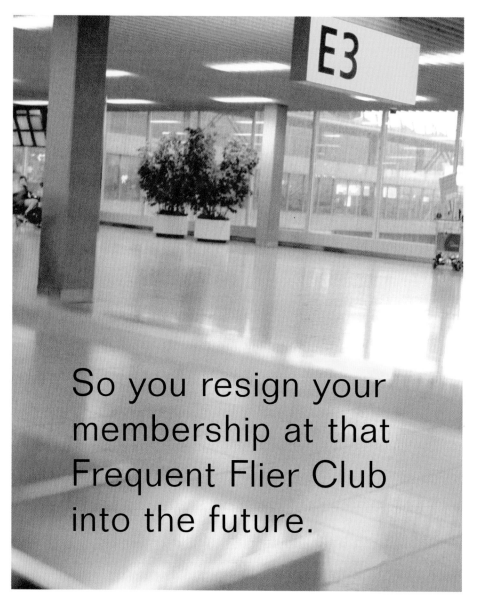

So you resign your membership at that Frequent Flier Club into the future.

And you ban those rousing Frequent Flier Club Cheerleading Chants, like:

1- "I'm worried that..."

2- "I can't until..."

3- "Someday I will..."

4- "What if..."

5- "I'll have another scotch on the rocks..."

Which brings you to...

LIFE LESSON

#21

You must remember:

You are here now...no, no, NOW...

no, now!

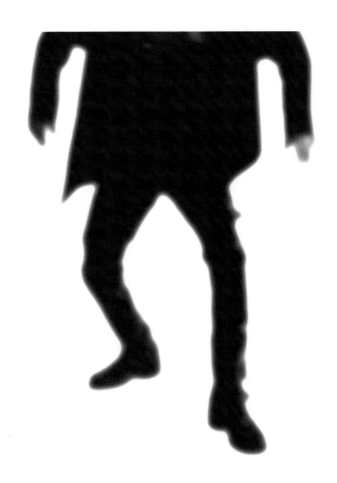

You are a human being and not a human was or a

human will be.

So you try to spend more
time being present —
and less time being busy.
Though granted, things
have gotten a heck more
hectic since you were
born. You now even have
an answering machine.
(You now even have
people to avoid on this
answering machine.)

You also know that sometimes you can get so outrageously busy that you could pass by a troll standing on the street corner waving a million bucks at you...

and you might not even notice.

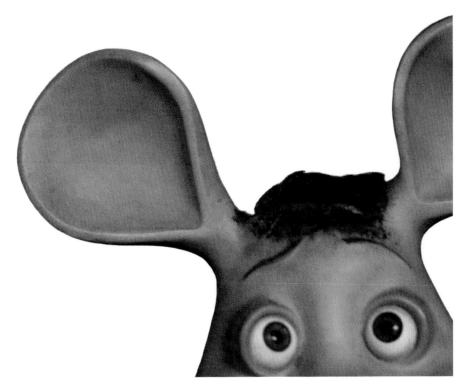

#22

It doesn't matter how fast you get there, if you're heading in the wrong direction.

So...you must slow down and see where you are going, buddy!

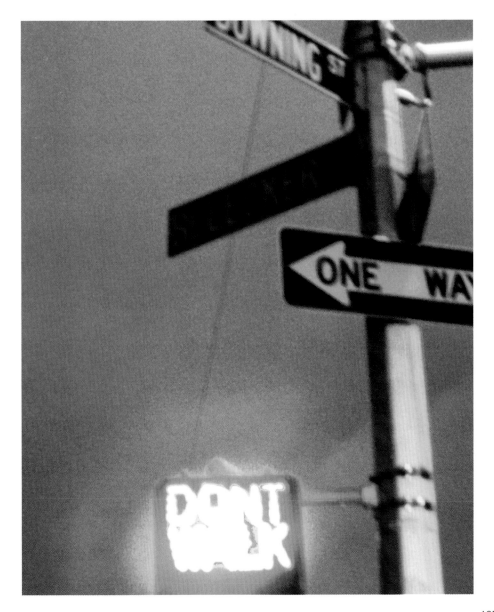

Though you think instead of
calling it "slowing down" it
should be called "slowing up,"
because when you take your
time...you save time.

"Slowing Up" (a quickie explanation):

It means you do not live in the past (with old habits), nor in the future (with not-so-great expectations), but here, in the moment — where the true you — and your true power — and the true answers to your problems — can all be found.

Which reminds you of yet another little story.

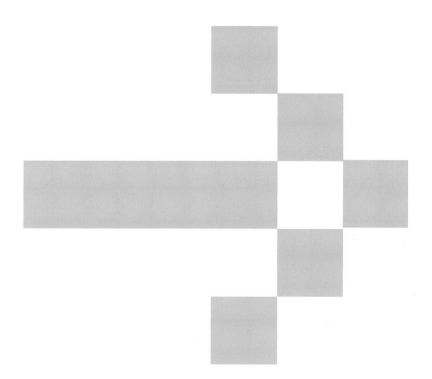

"I'm Dancing as Slowly as I Can"

You remember back to a dance class you took at your gym. The teacher showed you this complicated dance that you were expected to learn by hour's end. You remember thinking: "Yeah right, lady." But then she slowed down the music — played it at a much slower tempo — so you could see the steps weren't so mindboggling — or feetboggling. And sure enough within 60 minutes you were a regular Fred Astaire.

You know the same approach works for the complicated fancy footwork it takes to switch out of a bad relationship or a bad career. At first glance it looks like so much effort. Then when you relax you can see what the Buddhists see...

the 1,000-mile journey begins with one step.

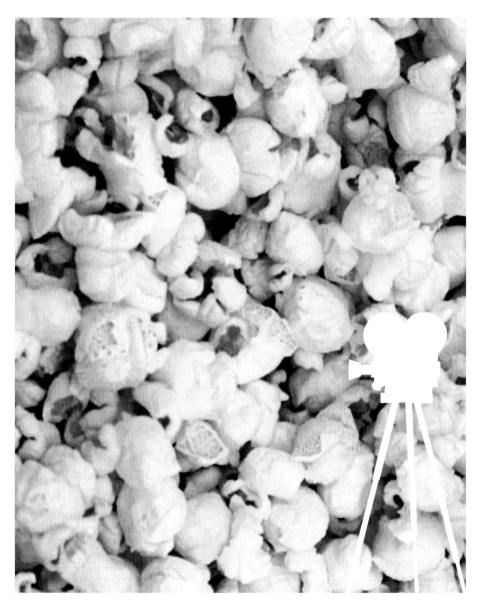

It's like how in the movies, folks like Clint or Sylvester or Sigourney know to remain cool and calm even when their futures look bleak and doomed. Although these people are often called "action heroes," you know their real power comes from being "still heroes," masters of the art of staying still within — of being fully, deeply present.

The Buddhists call this
mindfulness.

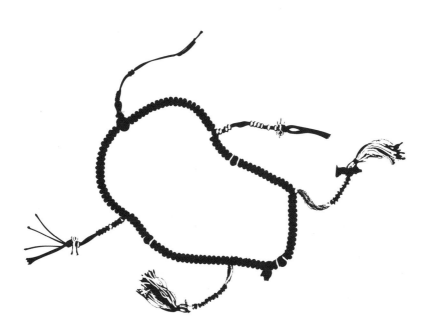

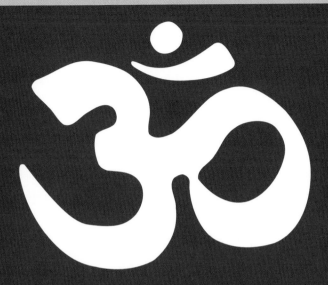

Though in many ways it's like mind-unfullness because it is all about entering into an empty-mind state, void of worries and fears and insecurities...a state that can be best achieved through regular meditation.

Which brings you to...

LIFE LESSON

When you practice regular meditation, you find you are able to see so much more.

#23

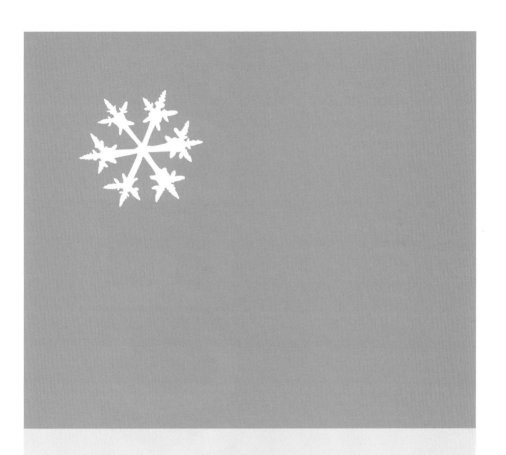

Meditation works like one of those shake-up-snow-dome thingies —
it helps the flaky stuff in your mind settle down, so you can see more
clearly what you truly need and want.

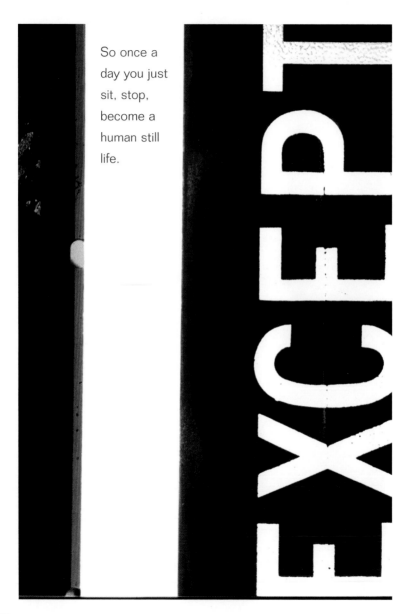

So once a day you just sit, stop, become a human still life.

Do nothing.
Be nothing.

Except breath. You become at one with your breath. You breathe. In and out. In and out. In and out. You shhhhhh and ignore the shhhhh*t.

You've found that once you've opened your eyes from meditation, that's when you see stuff like...

Whaddayaknow...

That chain around your leg is attached to a teeny-weeny twig.

Whaddayaknow...

You are really an eagle who longs to soar in the sky. All you have to do is flap!

Which brings you to...

LIFE LESSON

#24

When you become calm and serene on the inside, the world becomes more calm and serene on the outside.

You find that when you meditate more, you make better choices more — find better people more — and better opportunities more. So much so... it feels almost like magic!

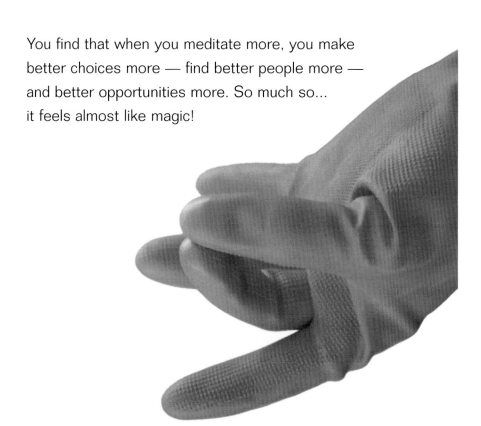

Some may call this good fortune "synchronicity." Some may call it "luck." Some may call it "intuition." Some may call it Ralph. (Admittedly very few people, though.) Some may call it "tapping into the collective unconscious."

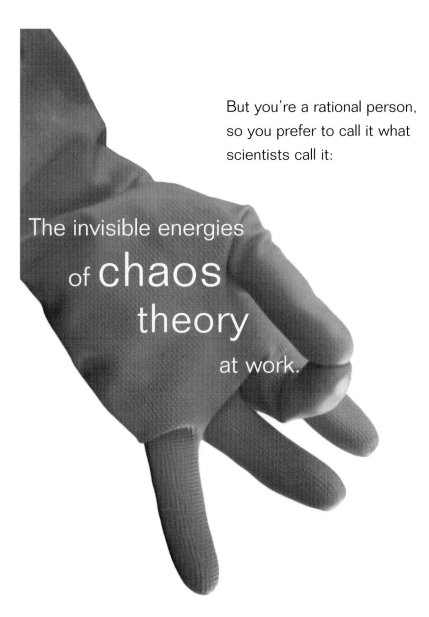

But you're a rational person, so you prefer to call it what scientists call it:

The invisible energies of chaos theory at work.

Which brings you to...

LIFE LESSON

#25

You must understand that there is chaos in this
world — as well as order in all chaos. In the same
way there's order in a seemingly chaotic subway
station, there's order in all the chaos of life around
you. The trick is to try to see the order in your
chaos, and to accept that...

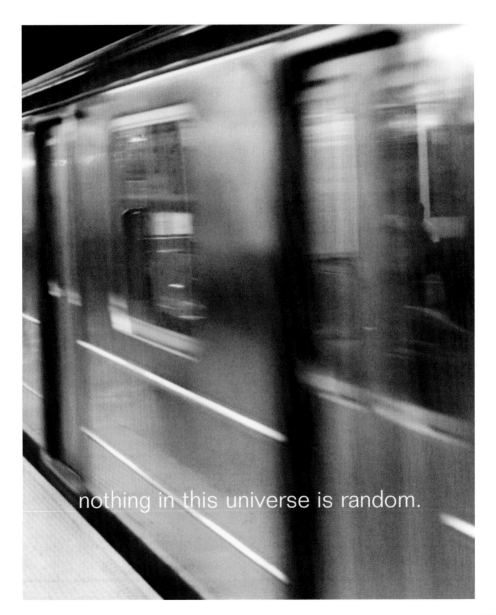

nothing in this universe is random.

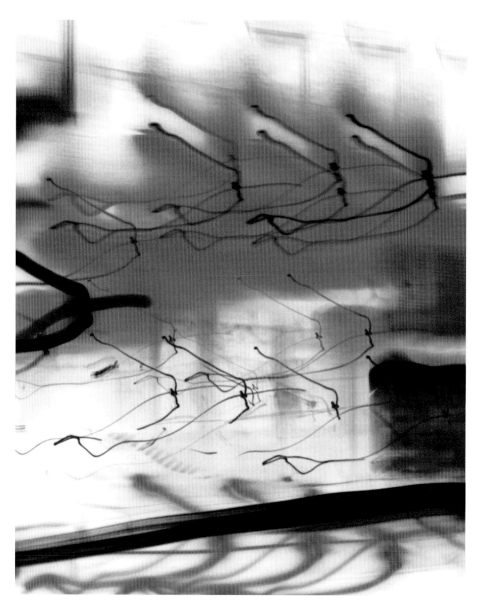

Both form and formlessness are connected within the same vibrating field all around you. All molecules are energy — and all energy is in motion at varying speeds — all around you, at all times.

Some molecules vibrate at slower speeds — and those vibrating at very slow speeds are what you presently perceive as the material world. And those molecules vibrating at hyper-fast speeds are the invisible energy of your thoughts.

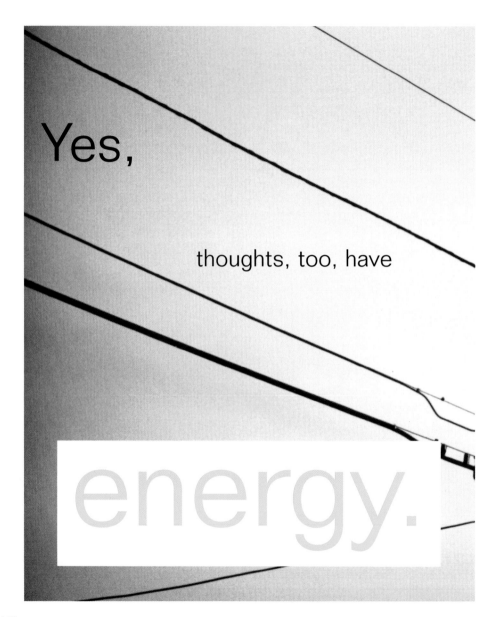

Yes,

thoughts, too, have

energy.

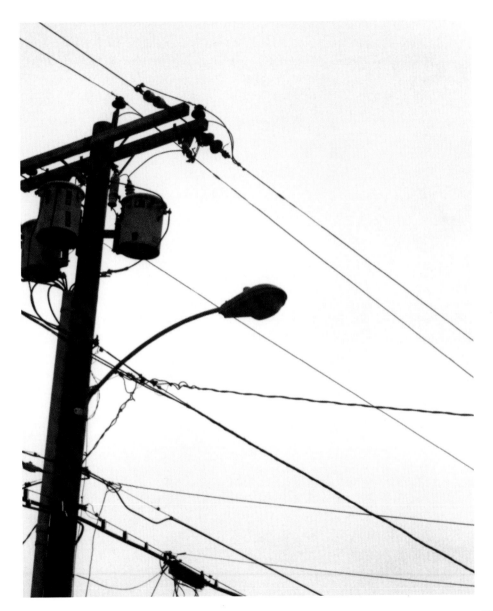

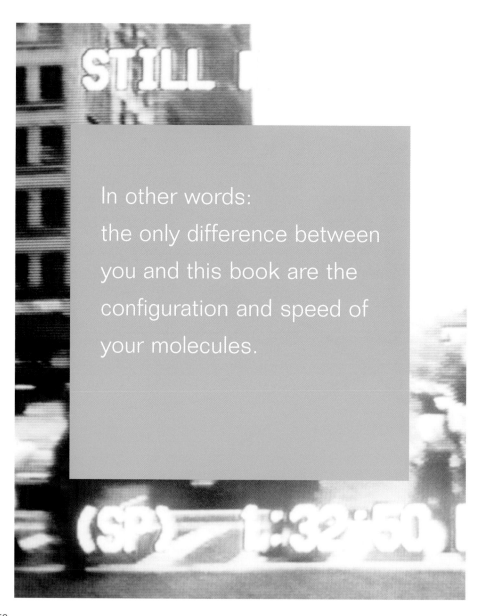

In other words:
the only difference between
you and this book are the
configuration and speed of
your molecules.

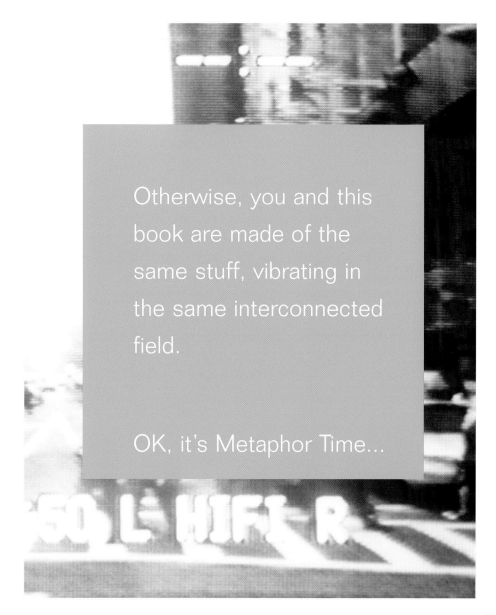

Otherwise, you and this book are made of the same stuff, vibrating in the same interconnected field.

OK, it's Metaphor Time...

"Field Goals"

You are like a tiny fish surrounded by a field of water but unable to see this water. What's going on in this field around you sends out waves that affect you. Likewise, what you do — and think — sends out waves into this field around you. This includes your negative thoughts — which can create distracting tidal waves that block you from seeing how to best get to your goal.

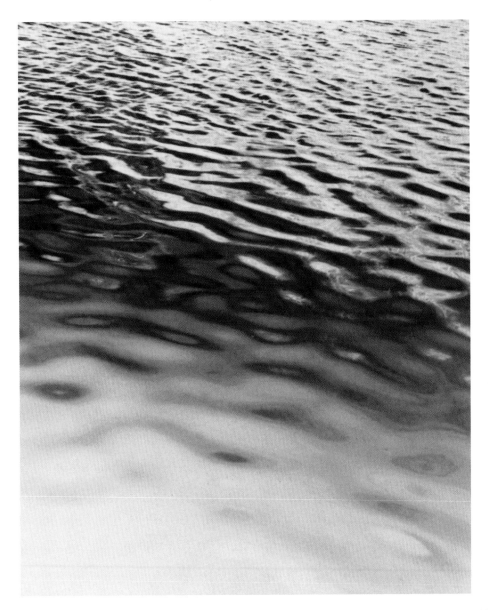

(huh?)

the explanation:

You are like a tiny fish surrounded and connected to the energy field that originated from that pot of Bubbling Primordial Stew. You — yes, lil' ol' you — are connected to all the infinite knowledge found in this original macro Primordial Stew ocean.

The explanation of the explanation: If you shift your awareness from the ordinary — which can be done through meditation as well as basic relaxation — you can sense this infinite, invisible, vibrating, all-knowing energy that is within you and around you, and can tap into that stuff that some call intuition, some call synchronicity, some call Ralph.

The explanation of the explanation of the explanation: When you are calm within, you can better see the order in the chaos — almost as if you have been given a secret map of this chaos that shows you the paths you need to take to get where you need to go!

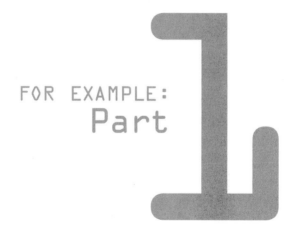

FOR EXAMPLE:
Part 1

This infinite, invisible, vibrating, all-knowing energy is what dogs tap into when they sense an earthquake coming.

And what moms tap into when they sense that their distant baby is in danger.

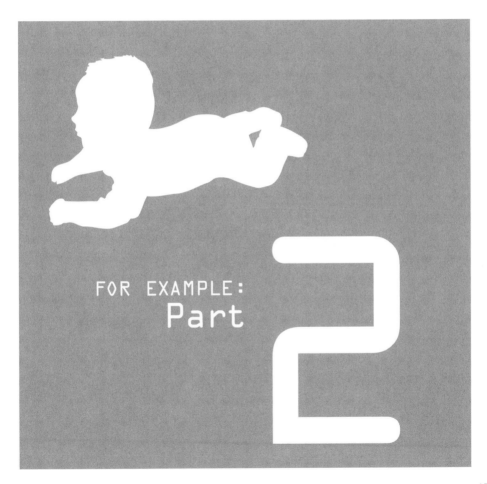

FOR EXAMPLE:
Part

2

And what you tap into when you think of a person and then they call you moments later.

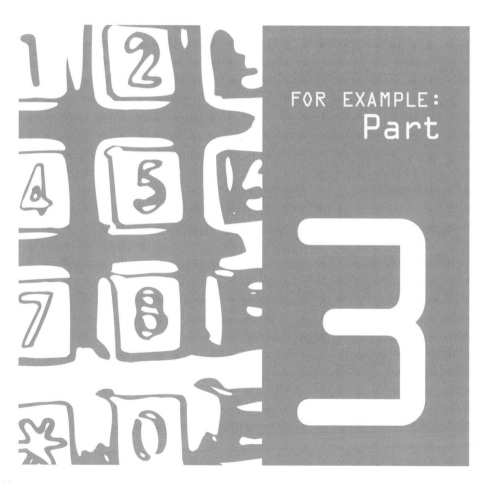

FOR EXAMPLE:
Part

3

FOR EXAMPLE:
Part

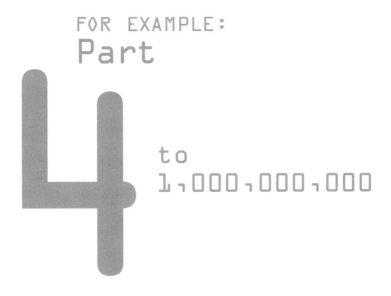

to
1,000,000,000

And what you tap into when you meet the very type of person that you have in your head that you've been needing to meet — in business and/or love, etc., etc.

Once and for all...

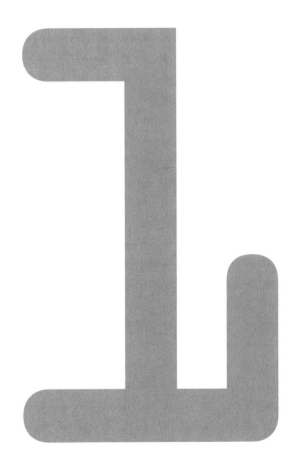

All is one.

You know: all of this sounds

weird,

freaky,

psychedelic,

man.

You also know: it explains a lot of the weird, freaky, psychedelic, man things that have happened to you.

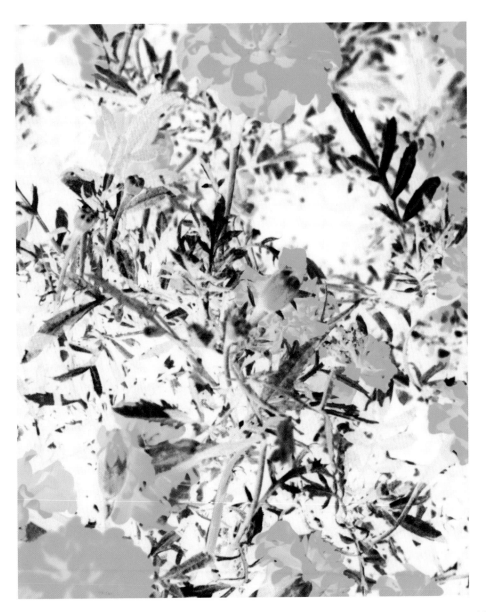

Which brings you to...

#26

You must show more

respect

for the invisible world,
because often what
you don't see is what
you get.

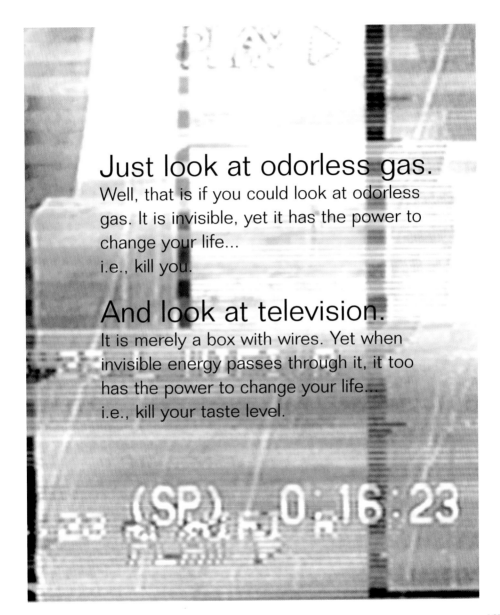

Just look at odorless gas.
Well, that is if you could look at odorless gas. It is invisible, yet it has the power to change your life...
i.e., kill you.

And look at television.
It is merely a box with wires. Yet when invisible energy passes through it, it too has the power to change your life...
i.e., kill your taste level.

And look at harmonic resonance — which you can look at, on any two guitars. When an "E" string is plucked on one, it will resonate on the other. You believe harmonic resonance works with people, too. When you speak openly from your heart, the hearts of others seem to open. This is because you are helping the people around you to vibrate at your same higher harmonic level. You've heard this called "companion energy." And you believe that in the same way the invisible germs of a cold can be contagious, or the invisible oxygen dynamics of a yawn can be contagious, the invisible energy of thoughts are contagious.

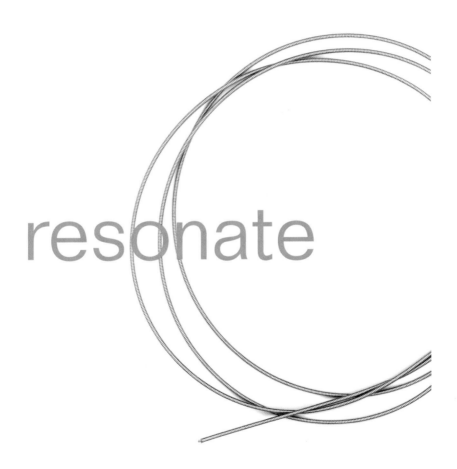

resonate

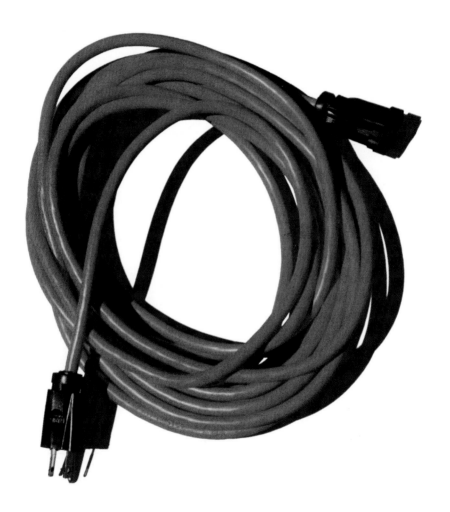

Your Local Quantum Physicist has even documented how the brain has electrical energy that gives off varying vibrations depending upon thoughts and mood. Because like energy attracts like energy, it makes sense that positivity might indeed attract positive results — even "positive, lucky coincidences."

You believe this may also explain why the rich get richer, why misery loves company, and why whenever you've already got a paramour it's way easier to get a paramour.

And this is also why fear attracts fear. Like your fear of not being able to fall asleep always seems to attract the problem of your not being able to fall asleep. Ditto for your fear of falling in love. Ditto for your fear of being too successful.

Which brings you to...

LIFE LESSON # 27

Worry and doubt can actually be prayers
and visualizations — and self-fulfilling
programming — for things you do not want.

self-

fulfilling programming

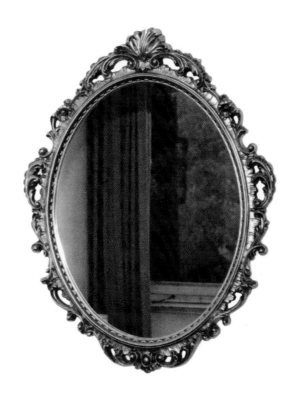

The world is your mirror.

Everything is created twice. What you have running in the programming of your mind eventually manifests itself in the outer world.

So if you want to change your outer world, you must first change your internal mental programming. When you try to change the external world first, it's like trying to change the picture on a TV screen by rubbing that picture with a cloth. You can rub, and rub, and rub — but it's futile, baby.

However...when you change your mental programming — who you are thinking you are and what you are thinking you deserve — you find the world around you changes simultaneously.

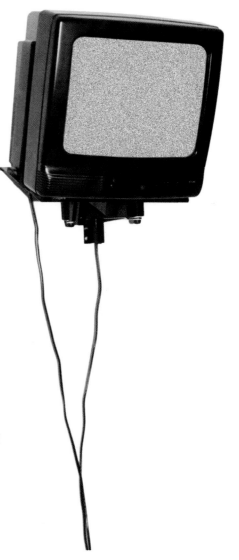

Which brings you to...

#28

Chaos Theory affects you daily —

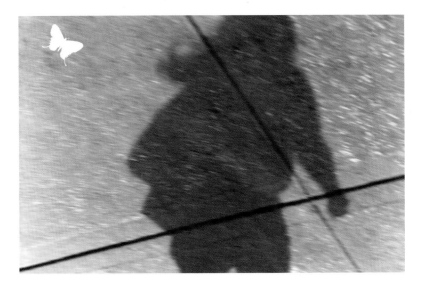

from the turbulence of today's weather to the complicated beatings of your heart, to all sorts of assorted areas in your life. The theory states that there is order and pattern where you might think there is only randomness and unpredictability. One of the most talked about principles of Chaos Theory — The Butterfly Effect — goes so far as to say that even the tiniest action can set off a chain of larger reactions — like the mere fluttering of a butterfly's wings in New York can transform storm systems in Tibet next month.

And the tiniest actions can also create reactions within your brain, heart, and body. Your Local Neurologist has even documented how the "action" of the mere twitch of a smile can set off the "reaction" of a stream of happy endorphins throughout your body. It seems the smile forces certain facial muscles to contract, which decreases the flow of blood in nearby vessels, which cools the blood, which lowers the temperature of the brain stem, which then produces more of a neurotransmitter called serotonin — which then puts you in a perkier mood.

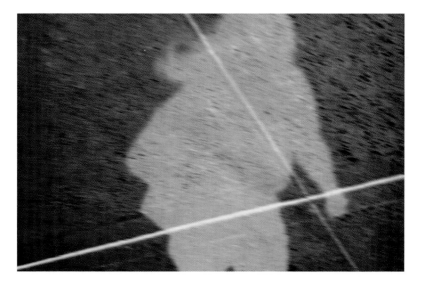

Plus your Local Neurologist has also documented how a person who is happy is better able to retrieve happy thoughts/ideas from their brain because these information bits are simmering at similar temperatures.

Which leads you to...

#29

There's great power in: I Think Therefore I Have.

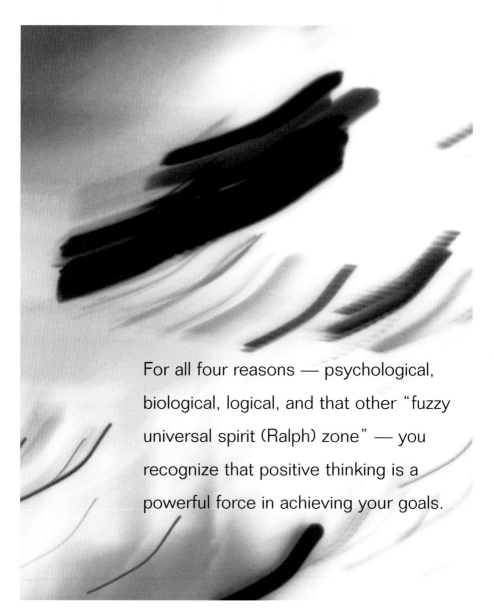

For all four reasons — psychological, biological, logical, and that other "fuzzy universal spirit (Ralph) zone" — you recognize that positive thinking is a powerful force in achieving your goals.

So, you decide to follow A Positive Thought Diet Program:

You start your day by reminding yourself how you are the type of person who attracts the thing/quality/love you want. You end your day by looking for the positive things you've brought toward you (in a similar way to when you are waiting in a long, long movie line, you look at how far you've come, rather than at the hopelessly long line ahead). And...speaking of waiting time...you use yours (waiting for movies, elevators, buses, call-waiting) to repeat positive thinking mantras.

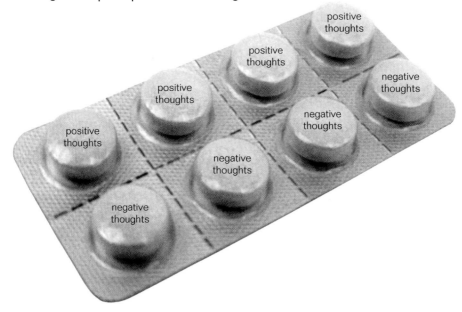

You make a list of all the reasons why you're worthy to get this thing/quality/love you want — and fully convince yourself of it.

You clip photos from magazines of your goal, and keep them nearby for an emotional boost.

You remind yourself of all the other times you've gotten the thing/quality/love you want — which means you can do it yet again!

Then...you do ditto for how others have achieved their goals.

You transform any negative jealousy into positive inspiration — as proof that what you want can be gotten!

You exercise and eat healthy foods so as to keep your mental attitude up and perky.

You recognize that mind and body are one — except during PMS, when mind and body are about 2 1/2.

You keep in mind what Ralph Waldo Emerson said about the mind: "A man becomes what he thinks about most of the time." (In other words, you can fall prey to the ol' "I think...therefore I am depressed.")

Whenever you're feeling pissed off or pissed on, you grab for a positive thought and use it as an emotional jack to get your spirit up and running smoothly. Plus, you jump-start positive endorphins by reading something funny — or seeing a funny movie.

Or...you write a list of 10 funny interpretations of that something bad in your life.
Or...you retrain your mind not to focus on this bad thing at all, but rather on the 9 great things happening.
Or...if you only have one great thing happening, you refocus on this, knowing even if it's a tiny positive thing — a little teeny-weeny ember of positivity — if you fan this ember it will grow.

You know this Positive Thought Diet Program will shape up your life if followed — as long as it's followed regularly.

Which brings you to...

#30

You cannot expect to see results from your Positive Thought Diet Program unless you follow it consistently and over time.

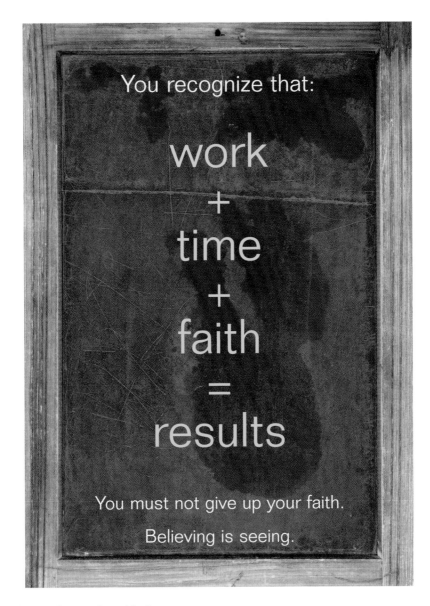

You recognize that:

work

+

time

+

faith

=

results

You must not give up your faith.

Believing is seeing.

Which reminds you of an old joke...

"H2-Uh-Oh"

A man was drowning in the ocean, hoping maybe God might save him. Soon, a small boat rowed up and offered to help him, but he, still testing to see if God would save him, sent the boat away. Next, a big yacht came by and offered to help him, but he sent this yacht away, again testing to see if God would save him. Next, a helicopter flew by and offered to throw down a ladder, but the man sent this helicopter away, still holding out for God to save him. Soon after, he drowned. When this man got up to heaven, he asked God why He didn't save him? God explained, "Who do you think sent the boat, the yacht, and the helicopter?"

YOU KNOW: You're being sent boats, yachts, and helicopters all the time. You just have to jump on board. Actually, this is also the divine principle behind the ordinary story of a girl ultimately marrying the boy next door — how/why/when she finally notices he's right next door.

IN OTHER WORDS: If you want to find a loving, sexy, communicative soul mate, you have to first believe in the existence of such a creature, so you can recognize this creature when it walks by — and not to give up on your search.

AND IN SOME MORE WORDS: If you believe a building exists, then even if you get lost on your way to finding it, you'll keep driving because you know it exists. And you know what you're looking for.

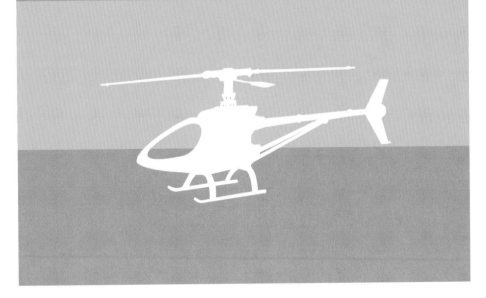

Which brings you to...

#31

Your faith determines your destiny.
So you must make sure your faith
remains stronger than your mood.

You must resist the temptation of giving up when your
hoped-for goal doesn't seem to be showing up! Which
reminds you of a quote from that underappreciated
Zen Philosopher, Bazooka Joe: "Your success is
limited only by your desire." You realize: Joe is
right — and pretty deep for a
bubble gum guy. In fact,
Bazooka Joe has given you
another juicy piece of
philosophy you often find
yourself chewing on...

LIFE LESSON # 32

"Never compromise your dreams,"
Bazooka Joe has said.

Joe's quote reminds you of another famous quote:
"The greatest enemy of the great is the good."
And what is "the good"? Another way of saying
"the choice you accept because you are afraid of
pursuing — or have given up on pursuing —
a greater choice."

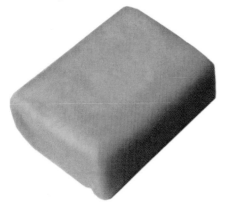
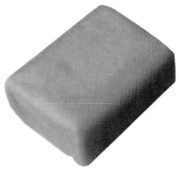

Which reminds you of an old Groucho Marx joke...

Groucho Marx was talking to a friend about marrying an unattractive mate, because a beautiful one could leave you. His friend reminds him: "An ugly one could leave you too." Groucho agrees, but explains, "Yeah, but if they do, who cares?"

You hear that joke and you know: you don't want to be a Groucho Marxist when it comes to compromise.

You want to resist settling for second best, or third best, or 127th best, when your #1 choice seems scary or slow in coming.

You see: if you cowardly settle for only the 5s life gives you (in lovers, friends, jobs, shoes, etc.), then you won't live a 10 life. Even if you gather a million 5s (i.e., a million 5-level lovers), because you'll still be creating a median of a 5 life. Not the 10 life you want. Not the satisfying life you want.

You realize: this is also why sometimes after you get a 5 something — you do not want that 5 something — because it is the wrong something — selected by the fearful, insecure 5-esque something inside you — that pesky 5-esque phantom of your 5-dom past, who holds you back with those convictions that life can only come in one 5-osity flavor.

You know: you must let go of those 5s.

Which brings you to...

LIFE LESSON

#33

When you let go of unnecessary attachments, you pick up speed in heading toward your true goals.

For this reason, it's always better to have a short bad relationship than a long bad relationship. Or a short unsatisfying career versus a long unsatisfying career.

190

The sooner the eagle flies the coop, the sooner the high-flying eagle livin' begins. Though you also know it's scary to

let go.

What if you fall?
What if you don't have eagle wings after all — and cannot fly?

Which brings you to...

You must live your life using the same philosophy a mountain climber uses to climb a mountain: "Never look down. Keep looking forward and upward."

LIFE LESSON # 34

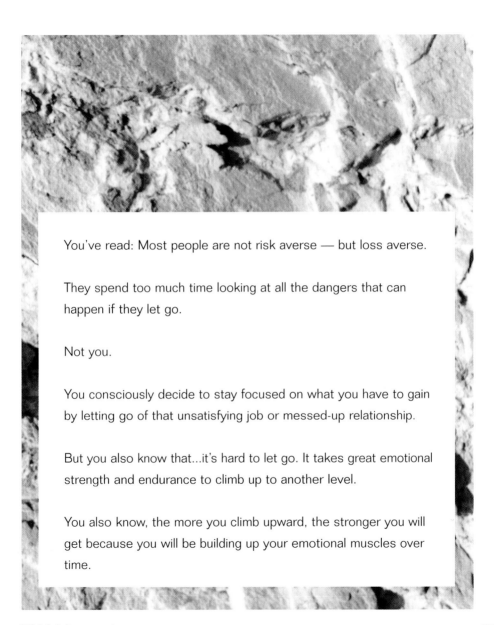

You've read: Most people are not risk averse — but loss averse.

They spend too much time looking at all the dangers that can happen if they let go.

Not you.

You consciously decide to stay focused on what you have to gain by letting go of that unsatisfying job or messed-up relationship.

But you also know that...it's hard to let go. It takes great emotional strength and endurance to climb up to another level.

You also know, the more you climb upward, the stronger you will get because you will be building up your emotional muscles over time.

Which brings you to...

LIFE LESSON

#35

Letting go and climbing up to higher life levels, means building new emotional muscles. And just like with all muscle growth, you will always feel the pain before you see the growth.

You've felt this pain first hand — and first heart. Like the last time you broke up with an unsatisfying paramour...in hope of finding a highly satisfying paramour. It was not until much later that you realized this pain did lead to your emotional growth.

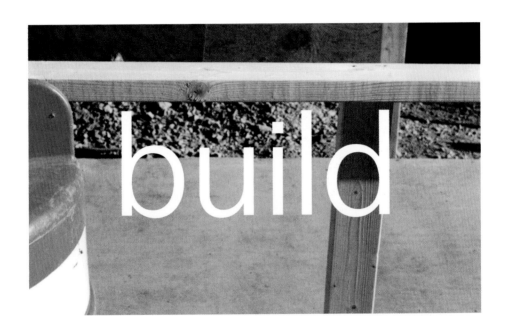

It just took time, dammit.

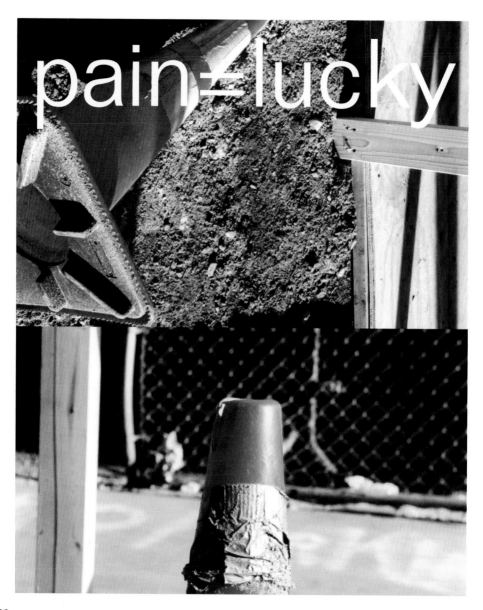

pain≠lucky

So you remind yourself to remind yourself
that next time you feel emotional pain that
you are lucky. You are getting stronger.
Things are improving — although you
might not see it right away. It's like when
your home was being painted and it looked
its utmost worst. Total chaos. However,
underneath this chaos was renovation in
motion. And because you were aware that
this painting action was leading to a more
beautiful home, you could relax, breathe
easily, accepting the chaos around you.
Same goes with your life.

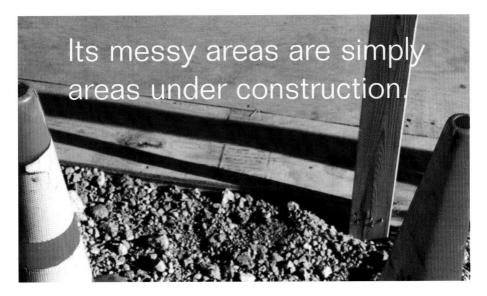

Its messy areas are simply
areas under construction.

Which brings you to...

#36

Everything has its process.

You must respect this process.

Just like with the painting process, your life improvement process can't be rushed.

Which reminds you of something very deep and wise your painter told you as he headed out the door midday for pizza: "You can't paint over a wet coat," he said. "You gotta wait for it to dry, otherwise you keep painting and painting and you get nowhere, you know?"

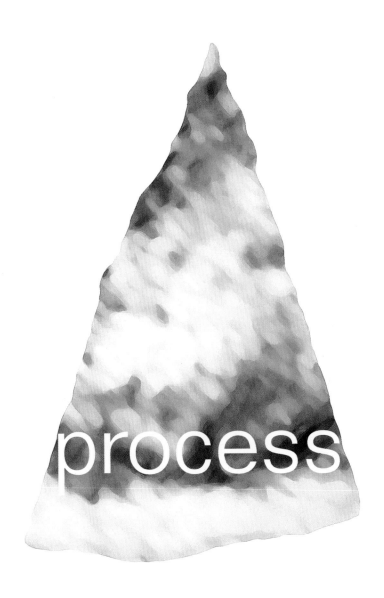

process

Which leads you to...

#37

Often doing less, gets you more.

Truly:

less

is more...more or less.

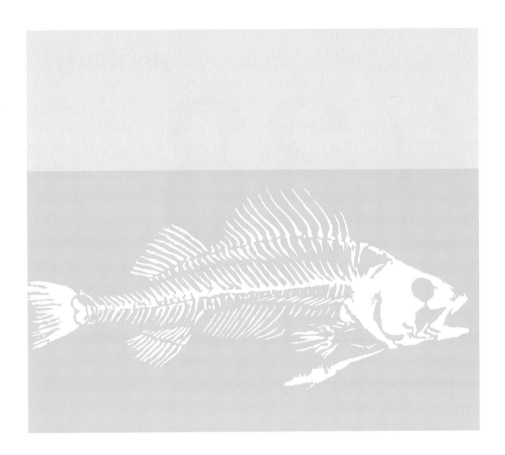

Getting what you want does not always mean hard work and struggle. Often, it's when you relax and stop resisting that what you want can't resist you. The Taoists advise about this: "Be careful not to turn over a fish too many times or it shall fall apart." However, the Taoists also believe in duality, meaning — the opposite of this is also true.

Which brings you to...

#38

You must create your own good luck. You must be pro-active — and even pre-active.

You must know when it's time to stop sitting around all relaxed, waiting for things to just happen to you — and instead stand up and take life by the shirt collar — and not be afraid to wrinkle that shirt collar. You alone decide on your own the level of love and money and happiness you attract to yourself.

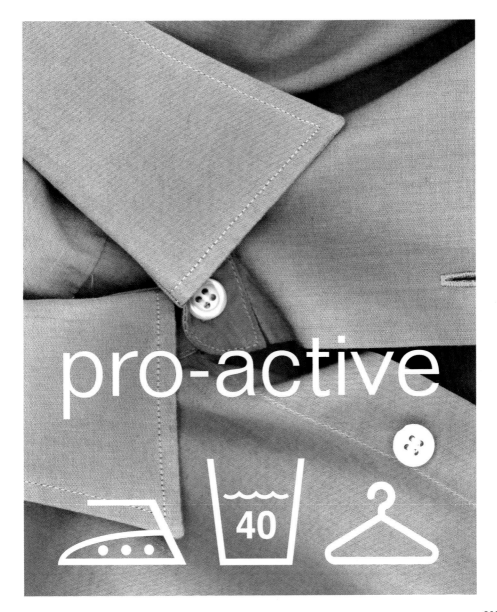

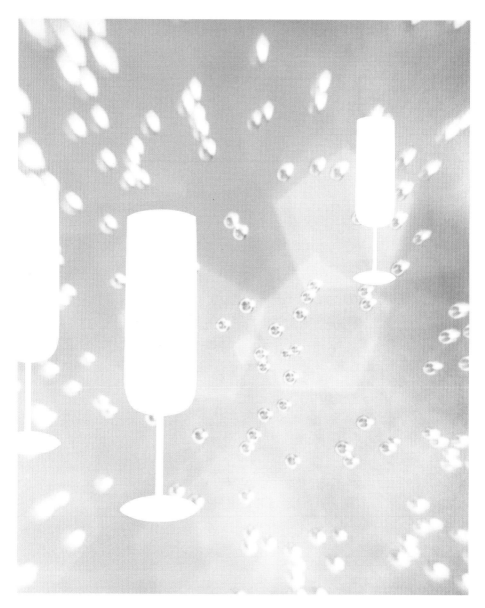

Or as Roseanne once said: "The thing women have got to learn is that nobody gives you power. You just take it." You know Roseanne is right. Whether you be a man or you be a woman — you are your own waiter in this cafe called Life. You decide what to serve yourself — the cheeseburgers of existence or the caviar and champagne treatment.

And although the aforementioned champagne was metaphysical champagne, you also know what you need to know when it comes to indulging in that real good materialistic champagne stuff.

Which brings you to...

39

Money will never bring you true happiness — however, happiness will bring you true money.

Expensive champagne will never be the panacea for extensive emotional pain. However, if you are happy doing what you are doing, then that's when the money will surely come.

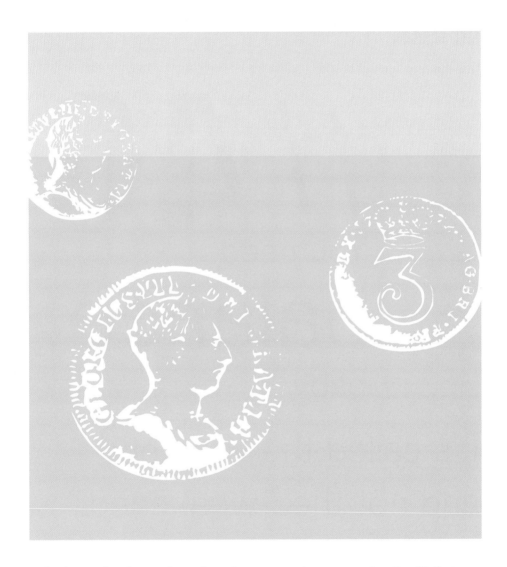

And you also know that when the money does come (as it will) that...

#40

You need
balance,
baby.

It's called the weekend —
and not the "weakened."

It's not "he who dies with the most toys wins." It's "he who has the most time to play with his toys and the most fun playing with them who wins." In other words: all work and no play means a life of all ego and no spirit.

True success is not about making lots of moola so you can get yourself expensive toys for your ego — nor is it about getting yourself a cute, sexy person for your ego. True success is about satisfying your spirit with spirit things. For instance, your ego looks at a cute, sexy person and says, "Yum, yum. I want that person." But your spirit is smarter. It looks at loving, joyous couples and thinks, "Mmmm, I want that joy, that happiness, that love."

Your spirit wisely knows: it's not a mate's superficial qualities that ultimately make you happy, but the dynamic this mate and you have together — and the blissful feelings this mate can give you in your true (and eagle) heart. Which reminds you of a lesson you learned reading *The Little Prince*: "It is only with the heart that one can see rightly; what is most important is invisible to the eye." And with this in mind — and heart — you decide to let this wise spirit of yours do all your

life shopping.

And with this in mind — and heart — you also decide: next time a paramour's not gonzo, then you're gone-zo. Because you now know: a paramour without love is merely an empty container. And who wants an empty container? The container is not the sustainer. You must not confuse the bottle for the juice. The bottle might satisfy your ego, but only the juice can feed your heart.

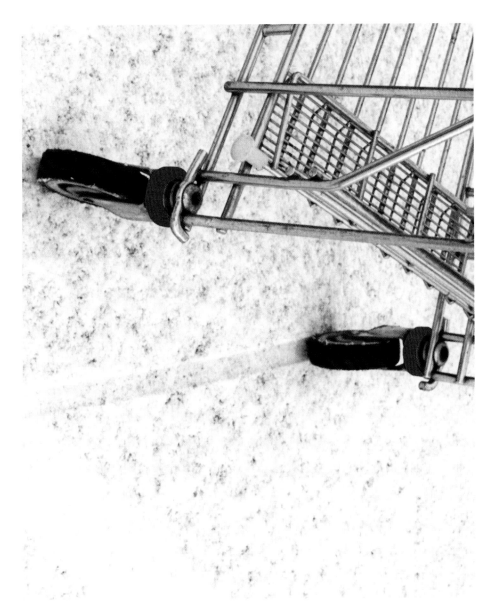

Which brings you to...

#41

Prozak Shmozak. Love Is the Drug.

Love is what you're always looking for in all the things you're looking for.

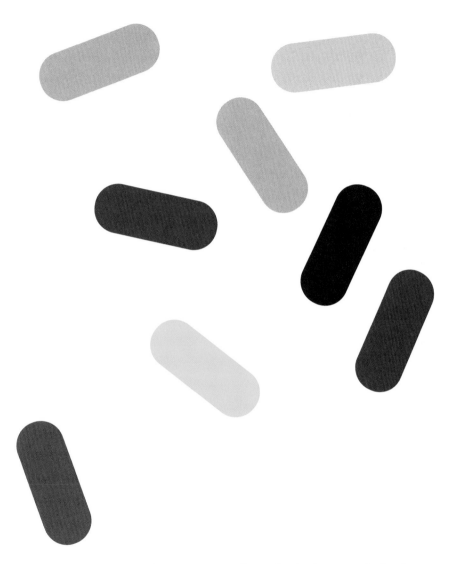

Even your yearning for sex is really a dyslexic search for love.

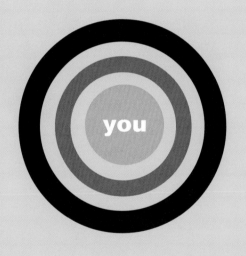

YOU KNOW IT.
AND AD AGENCIES KNOW IT.

Love is the #1 marketing strategy,
used as a promise in ad campaigns
for products from cars to toothpaste
to floorwax.

And all this Lovemania reminds you
of a Zen saying: "Basically the
archer aims at himself."

If you are not a happy person inside
you, then nothing outside you will
ever make you happy and able to
feel love.

This makes sense because you
know already from Lesson #27 how
the world is your mirror.

It thereby makes sense that if you
can increase how happy and loving
you feel about yourself on the
inside, the more happiness and love
you will see and attract from the
world around you to you.

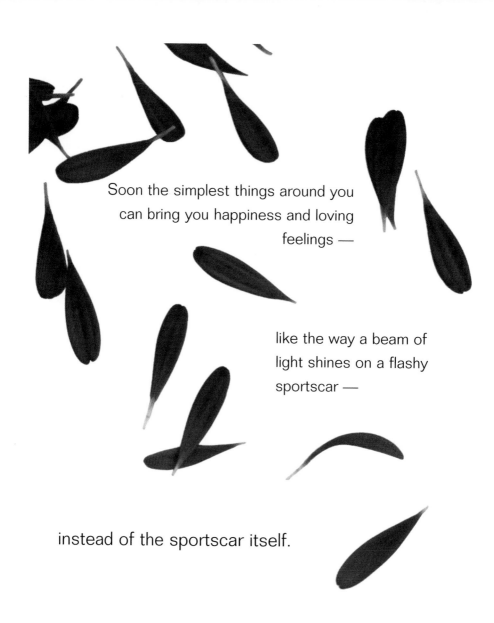

Soon the simplest things around you
can bring you happiness and loving
feelings —

like the way a beam of
light shines on a flashy
sportscar —

instead of the sportscar itself.

Or the sight of a perfect flower —
or an imperfect flower.

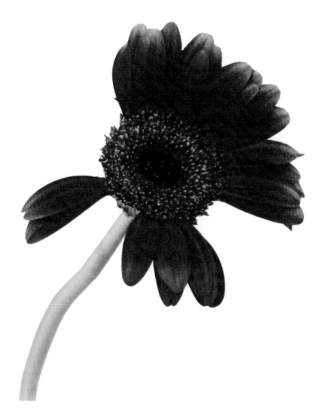

Which brings you to...

LIFE LESSON #42

Just like there's sexual attraction, there's love attraction. When you feel the love energy inside you, other people feel it coming off of you — and find themselves wildly — and oddly — attracted to you.

You've witnessed this yourself — how whenever you're in love you seem to attract more love to you — as well as other positive stuff. Yes, love is a boomerang, baby. What you have and give away is what you get back. Love energy attracts love energy — for the reasons you learned back in Life Lesson #26. It's all about "harmonic resonance" working its energies on those around you. And so with a fierce heart you work at attaining and maintaining this unconditional self-love for yourself and life within your fierce heart — and when you do, you see how life just loves the bupkiss out of you right back — and big time!

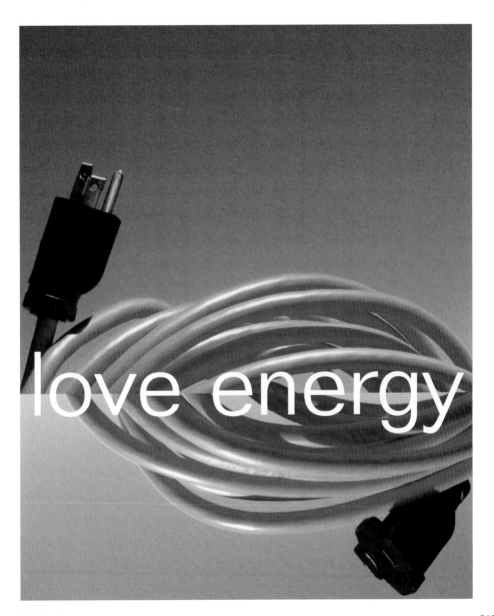

love energy

Which brings you to...

#43

LIFE LESSON

There's a

difference

between knowing vs. doing.

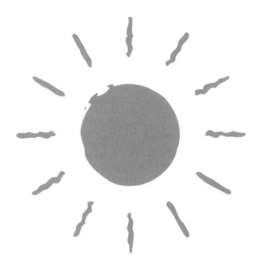

You know all of what is in this book is true —
and should be followed. Knowledge and ideas
are not enough. You must put in the effort and
discipline of action. You must truly live these
life lessons daily.

You must seize the day...

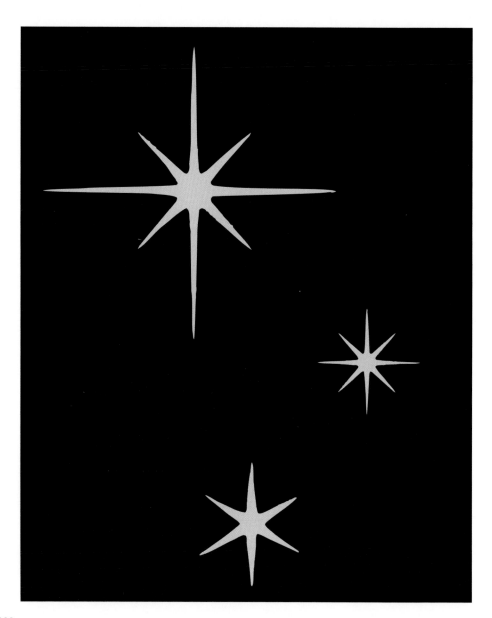

And seize the night...

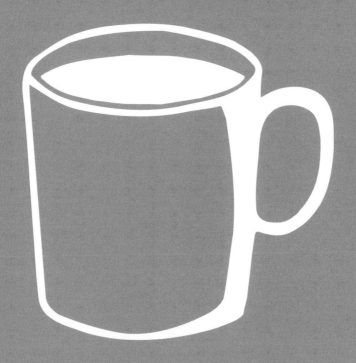

And seize the 3 o'clock coffee break.

You get the idea.
Seize it all.

What you seize is what you get.

Which all means...

#44

Live now,
procrastinate later.

What are you waiting for?
Start following this book now.

And we mean now, dammit.

Come on. We mean it.

Close the damn book already!

Scram.

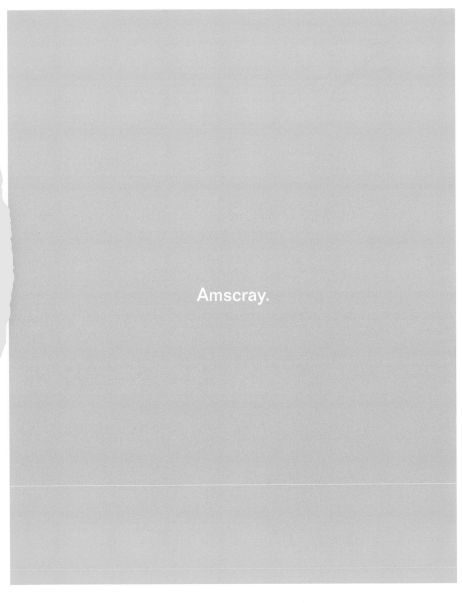

Amscray.

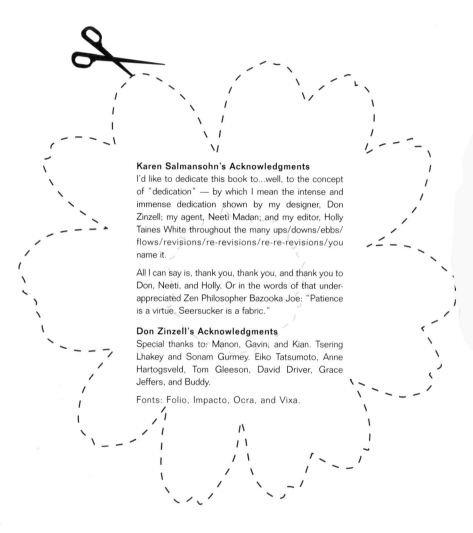

Karen Salmansohn's Acknowledgments

I'd like to dedicate this book to...well, to the concept of "dedication" — by which I mean the intense and immense dedication shown by my designer, Don Zinzell; my agent, Neeti Madan; and my editor, Holly Taines White throughout the many ups/downs/ebbs/flows/revisions/re-revisions/re-re-revisions/you name it.

All I can say is, thank you, thank you, and thank you to Don, Neeti, and Holly. Or in the words of that under-appreciated Zen Philosopher Bazooka Joe: "Patience is a virtue. Seersucker is a fabric."

Don Zinzell's Acknowledgments

Special thanks to: Manon, Gavin, and Kian. Tsering Lhakey and Sonam Gurmey. Eiko Tatsumoto, Anne Hartogsveld, Tom Gleeson, David Driver, Grace Jeffers, and Buddy.

Fonts: Folio, Impacto, Ocra, and Vixa.